Inner
Reiki

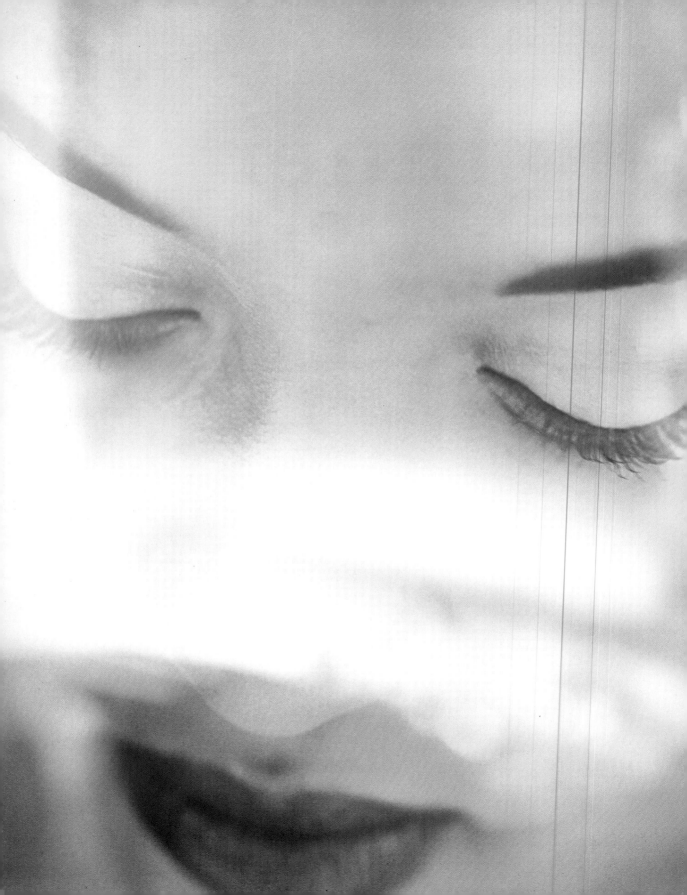

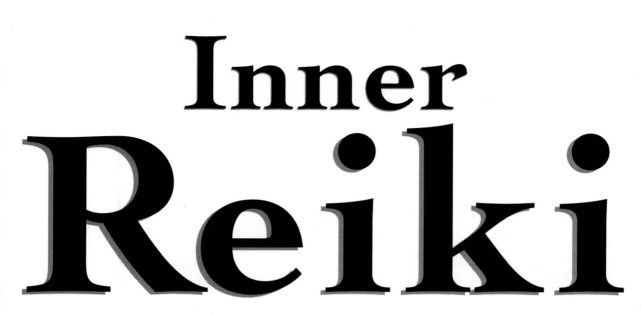

Inner Reiki

A Practical Guide for Healing and Meditation

TANMAYA HONERVOGT

An Owl Book
Henry Holt and Company
New York

Henry Holt and Company, LLC
Publishers since 1866
115 West 18th Street
New York, New York 10011

This book is dedicated to all human beings on planet earth, to encourage us to live in love, joy, and harmony, so that we can recognize the divine spark in each other.

You are the secret of God's secret.
You are the mirror of divine beauty.
Everything in the universe is within you.
Ask all from yourself,
The One at whom you are looking is also you.

Jelaluddin Rumi

Published in the United Kingdom in 2001 by Gaia Books Ltd.

Library of Congress Cataloging-in-Publication Data

Honervogt, Tanmaya.
Inner Reiki: a practical guide for healing and meditation/Tanmaya Honervogt —
1st American ed.
p. cm.
Includes index.
Originally published in London by Gaia Books Ltd.
ISBN 0-8050-6690-X(pbk.)
1. Reiki (Healing system) 2. Meditations. 3. Self-care, Health. I. Title.

RZ403. R45 H658 2001
615.8'52 – dc21   2001024540

Henry Holt books are available for special promotions and premiums.
For details contact: Director, Special Markets.

First Edition 2001

Designed by Phil Gamble

Printed and bound in Singapore by Kyodo

10 9 8 7 6 5 4 3 2 1

About this book

Reiki is a simple technique for transferring healing energy from a giver to a receiver. The word "Reiki" (pronounced "ray-key") means Universal Life Energy, and the ability to bring about healing during Reiki is gained through receiving attunements during a special initiation ceremony. The energy attunements open a channel in the giver for energy to flow through, to wherever it is most needed in the receiver. This can occur on a physical, mental, emotional, or spiritual level.

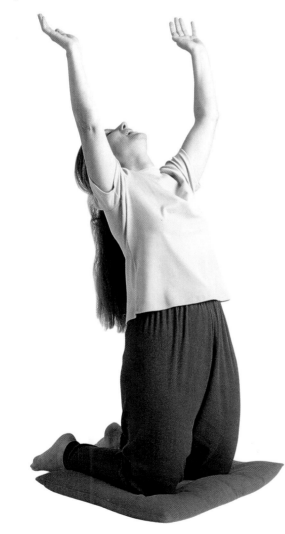

The attunements are transmitted during First, Second, and Third Degree trainings, by a certified Reiki Master-Teacher. The unique Reiki Symbols with their mantras, which enable the Reiki power to work on a vibrational level, are handed on from Reiki Master to student, in confidence, during the Second and Third Degree trainings. They are secret and are therefore not published in this book. However, the theory behind the use of the Symbols is fully explained and suggestions are made as to how each Symbol can be applied and used.

This book is intended for those who already have some knowledge of Reiki, but who want to deepen their experience of it by combining it with various forms of meditation. Thus Reiki becomes more personal and effective as a powerful healing tool.

CAUTION

The exercises, hand positions, meditations, and techniques described in this book are intended for the healing and harmonization of living things. The author nevertheless wishes to point out that, in the case of illness, a doctor or health practitioner should always be consulted. The Reiki positions described may naturally be applied as an additional form of treatment. Neither the author nor the publisher accept any responsibility for the application of the Reiki methods described in this book.

Contents

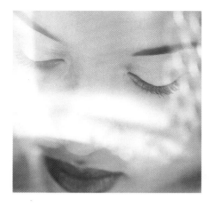

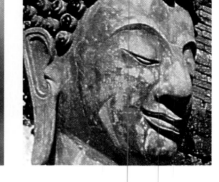

CHAPTER ONE
Reiki and meditation:
natural partners   12

CHAPTER TWO
Finding the mind-body
health connection   38

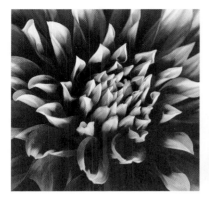
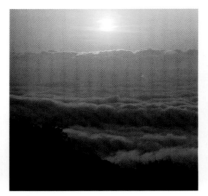
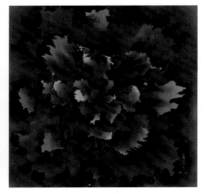

About the author

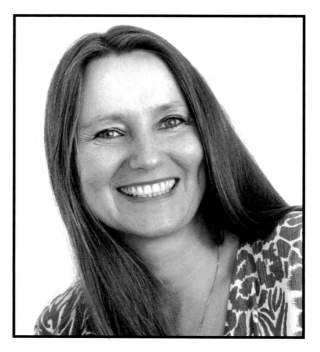

Tanmaya Honervogt is a Reiki Master–Teacher, healer, lecturer, author, and seminar leader. She spends her time between Germany and England, travelling extensively to Japan, Australia, USA, and throughout Europe, giving lectures and leading trainings. Since 1978 Tanmaya has been committed to her own self-development, studying and travelling as part of her quest, and integrating what she has learnt in her teaching skills, having originally trained as a school and language teacher. Out of the broad range of subjects she has studied, Reiki has become closest to her heart and she has been a practitioner since 1983, and Master since 1992. Underpinning Tanmaya's work is a path of meditation and all her Reiki trainings incorporate the flavour of meditation and reflect her own wisdom and understanding.

In 1981 Tanmaya met her spiritual master, Osho. His guidance and meditation techniques have since been a cornerstone in her life, which is shared in this book.

Tanmaya welcomes hearing from her students and readers and she is most easily contacted through the School of Usui Reiki website (www.school-of-usui-reiki.com) or by writing to PO Box 2, Chulmleigh, Devon, EX18 7SS, England, UK (please enclosed a stamped-addressed envelope). Tanmaya offers trainings and advanced courses in all three Reiki degrees all year. If you would like up-to-date information about her work, please write to the above address.

Introduction

Meditation is not a work, it is a play...
Meditation is not something to be done to
achieve some goal, peace, bliss. But something
to be enjoyed as an end in itself. The festive
dimension is the most important thing to be
understood, and we have lost it totally.
By festive I mean the capacity to enjoy
moment to moment
All that comes to you.

Osho, contemporary Indian mystic

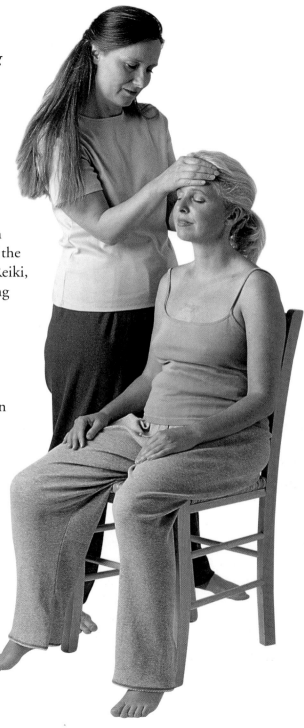

This book is about Reiki in combination with
meditation, each deepening the experience of the
other: meditation deepens the experience of Reiki,
and Reiki prepares you for meditation, relaxing
body, mind, and emotions. Since I have over
twenty years' experience as a meditator and
eighteen years' practising Reiki, it is my
experience that each can have the effect of
enhancing the other, allowing the individual
to go inside him- or herself, encountering even
deeper layers.

A DEEPER LEVEL

To learn Reiki you have to be open,
possessing a desire to become a channel for
healing energy to pass through you. Many
students also have a desire and a longing to
connect with themselves on a deeper level
and to get to know themselves better. My
main aim as a Reiki and meditation teacher
is to support this desire, and I know that
the two techniques provide the correct
tools for doing so. Over the past few
years of teaching Reiki, I have developed
advanced Reiki training, entitled *Inner Reiki:*

Reiki and Meditation. In these courses, which run over a weekend, students learn to bring meditation into their Reiki practice. This helps them to trust themselves more and it enhances their intuition.

IN TOUCH WITH INTUITION

When you are in touch with your intuition, you are in touch with something higher than yourself; higher than personality. Intuition is not logical; it is not connected with the rational mind or with conscious thinking. Rather, intuition comes from the superconscious mind, which is a higher level inside yourself.

THE NATURE OF THE SUPERCONSCIOUS

The superconscious is alert and full of light. It corresponds with the Higher Self, which knows and sees things clearly and gives you guidance through difficult and challenging periods of your life: for example, when you need to make an important decision about a change of job, moving house, or ending a relationship. To be able to trust your intuition and to connect to your Higher Self is an important skill to learn in life. Through this you receive inspiration, clarity, and courage to take the right decisions about necessary changes. Both Reiki and meditation strengthen this connectedness to your intuition and Higher Self and help you to trust your own insights and impulses. For example, when you are carrying out a Reiki treatment, your intuition can tell you where to place your hand on a receiver's body. You simply ask yourself, "Where are my hands needed right now?" and trust the first answer that springs into your mind.

CONTACTING THE CENTRE

During the course of a training weekend I introduce different meditation techniques and guide the student towards contacting his or her own centre. Before giving a Reiki treatment it is important to go inside and make contact with the centre, which is connected with the sacral (second) chakra, just below the navel. This is an area in the body where you can discover relaxation, rest inside yourself, and give yourself whatever nourishment you need. Through meditation you can relax completely and this will enhance your own process of healing, as well as deepening your meditation.

MEDITATION TECHNIQUES

There are different types of meditation technique, both active and passive. Active techniques usually have periods of physical activity and catharsis to unload any tension in the physical and emotional body. The Dynamic Meditation (see pp.64-7) is one such technique, developed by the Indian mystic Osho. This meditation technique allows you to express and deal with your emotions. Practising this meditation, you gain insight and ever-increasing awareness about yourself and become more silent and peaceful inside. Osho created methods of meditation specially for the modern man and woman and many of the meditation techniques featured in this book were developed by him.

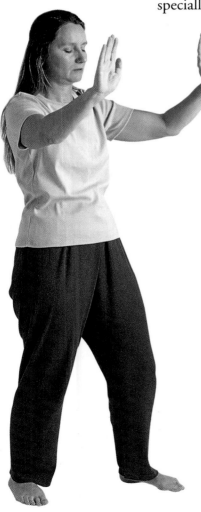

Out of this work and experience, I have been inspired to write this book.

I wish you love and light and further growth on your journey of self-exploration, remembering your divine connection; who you truly are — conscious awareness, a divine being of light.

Tanmaya Honervogt, February 2001

Chapter one

Reiki combined with meditation helps you to discover deeper layers within yourself and within the Reiki method. Reiki prepares you for meditation, and meditation deepens your experience of Reiki.

Reiki and meditation:

natural partners

Reiki is a gentle, powerful, hands-on healing technique. It is based on a specific energy attunement process (see p.118) in which ancient mantras and symbols are used to amplify the flow of life force energy and to open up the inner healing channel. This means that we use our natural ability to heal and allow more vital life force energy to flow through the upper energy centres (chakras). The energy then flows out through the arms and hands so that wherever we then place our hands healing energy is absorbed. Reiki revitalizes body, mind, and soul, relieves pain and stress, and helps in many conditions, always supporting the natural healing process.

HOW MEDITATION IS USED

Meditation is a precise, scientific way to go deeper within yourself. In this book meditation techniques are integrated into Reiki healing, allowing the Reiki giver and receiver to expand and grow in creative ways and to heal their own energy bodies. Old energy patterns can dissolve, energy centres become balanced, energy bodies are nourished, and the smooth flow of energy is re-established.

IMPORTANCE OF ACTIVE MEDITATIONS

Active meditations, where body movement is involved, are particularly important in lifestyles of today. We need to act out our energy, using the body to relax tension, and we need catharsis to unburden ourselves emotionally and mentally. If you are already a Reiki healer, you will find the active meditation techniques in this book invaluable for developing your healing power.

Meditation helps the flow of energy to expand – it starts to move upwards, affecting the etheric body (one of seven energy bodies) and its energy centres (the chakras). This brings silence whereas energy moving downwards causes tension.

Reiki energy opens up the space for healing and relaxation within; people frequently feel more contented and in touch with themselves after receiving it, commenting, "I feel as if I've done a meditation". They are at home in themselves and resting in their own centre.

Healing

Reiki is a perfect way of bringing healing to yourself and others, too. The Japanese character for healing lies behind the text on this page.

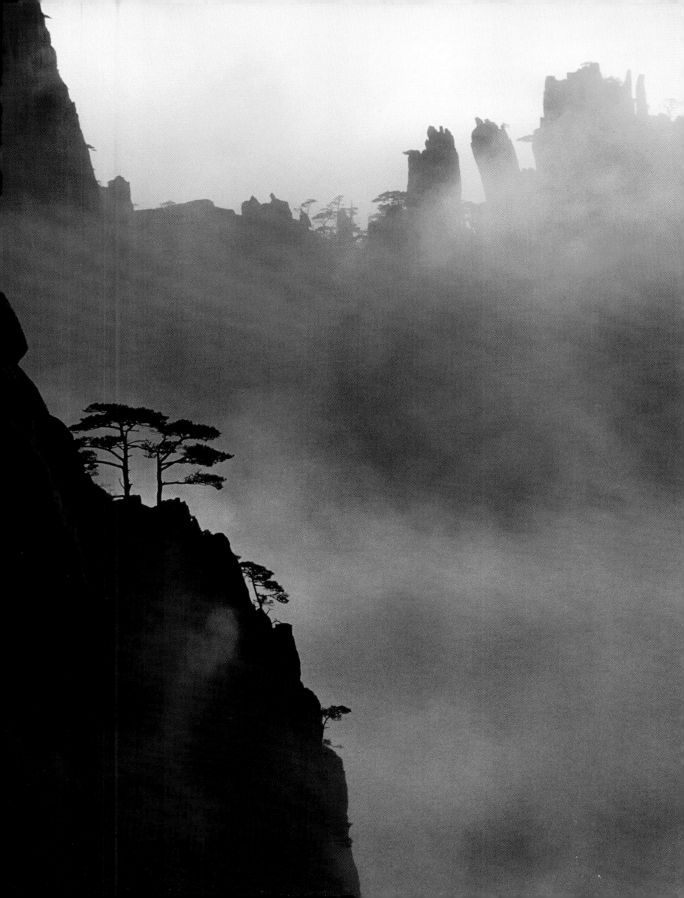

The effects of meditation

While you are sitting still in meditation, not doing anything, you have no "becoming", no desire; you just remain with yourself. You are silently witnessing what is happening and remaining in the centre, in yourself. So Reiki and meditation work together. Practising meditation techniques will help you to deepen your Reiki, while Reiki brings balance and harmony to all the different levels (physical, emotional, mental, and spiritual).

SELF-RELAXATION EXERCISE

Before you start to meditate, you first need to become fully relaxed. This exercise is to help you become aware of where you are holding tension in the physical body and to help you to relax the body–mind mechanism. It can revive childhood experiences, when you were so much more relaxed and full of energy.

Do this relaxation before going to sleep, or at any time of the day, over a few days. You give Reiki to your head while mentally focusing on other body parts. Play soothing music if you like.

Step one

Sit in a chair or lie down. Take a few deep breaths in through the nose and out through the mouth, making a little sigh with each out-breath. Feel your whole body relaxing and letting go of tension.

Step two

Now place your hands over your eyes, resting your palms on the cheekbones. After about 3 minutes, keeping your hands over your eyes, focus your awareness on your feet. Now start watching, with eyes closed, the energy coming up from your feet. Watch from inside to see whether there is tension in the feet. If you find tension try to relax your feet and don't move on from that point until you feel that relaxation has come.

Step three

Now move your attention to your legs and try to locate the tension there. Again, if you find tension, consciously relax there. Gradually focus awareness on all parts of your body. Move on to the groin area, belly, stomach, buttocks, hips, all the organs, lungs, shoulders, and arms. Work through your hands, which are connected with your mind. For example, if your left hand is tense, the right side of your brain is tense and vice versa.

Now relax your face and the skin of your head and neck. Watch any tension in your mind. Just by watching, the tension and thoughts disappear. When your whole body is relaxed your mind is relaxed, too.

The human energy field

Everything that is alive pulsates with energy. Practitioners of complementary medicine, as well as physicists, acknowledge the existence of an electromagnetic field generated by the body's biological processes. This energy field surrounding the physical body extends as far out as your outstretched arms and the full length of your body. It contains information and is a highly sensitive, perceptive system. Through this system, we are constantly in communication with everything around us and we transmit to, and receive messages from, other people's bodies as well.

A REFLECTION OF ENERGY

Alternative health practitioners, healers, and psychics believe that the human energy field contains and reflects each individual's energy. It surrounds us and carries the emotional energy created by our experiences, whether they are positive or negative. Experiences that carry emotional energy become accumulated in our energy system, including past and present relationships, profound and traumatic experiences, memories from past lives, our belief patterns, and the attitudes that we gather during upbringing. The emotions from these experiences become imprinted on our physical body and contribute to the formation of our cell tissue, which then generates a quality of energy that reflects those emotions.

ENERGY LANGUAGE

These energy impressions create an energy language carrying information that can be read by an intuitive practitioner, healer, or psychic. Think of an occasion when someone acknowledged you positively and praised you for something you did or for a creative achievement. You probably experienced a rush of positive energy, perhaps a surge of personal power and self-esteem, making you feel good about yourself. Positive images and experiences, as well negative

ones, are held in each energy field and they register a memory in the cell tissue and in the energy field. Our emotions live physically in our bodies and interact with our cells and tissues.

THE HUMAN AURA

The human energy field, usually called the "aura", can be described as an energy body that surrounds and interpenetrates the physical body. Researchers have created theoretical models that divide the aura into several layers. These layers are called "energy bodies", which interpenetrate and surround each other. Each successive body is composed of finer substances and higher vibrations than the body that it surrounds. Some people are able to "see" the aura and say that it is like a multi-layered energy field pulsating with colour, according to our mood and health.

CARING FOR OUR ENERGY BODIES

To keep our energy bodies healthy, we need to take good care of them. In order to do so we first need to become sensitive to their existence and to become aware of the ways in which they influence us. As we grow spiritually we become more sensitive to the energies around us. We feel and sense vibration and energy, and the more we learn how to purify and refine our own energy bodies, the more we notice the communication between other people's energy bodies. Our human task is to purify our energy bodies and give them the right kind of attention and nourishment. In this way we establish a harmony and growth between the different bodies that allows our energy to flow freely and keeps us healthy and balanced.

Visible colours
The various colours of the layers of the aura can be seen clearly in Kirlian photography.

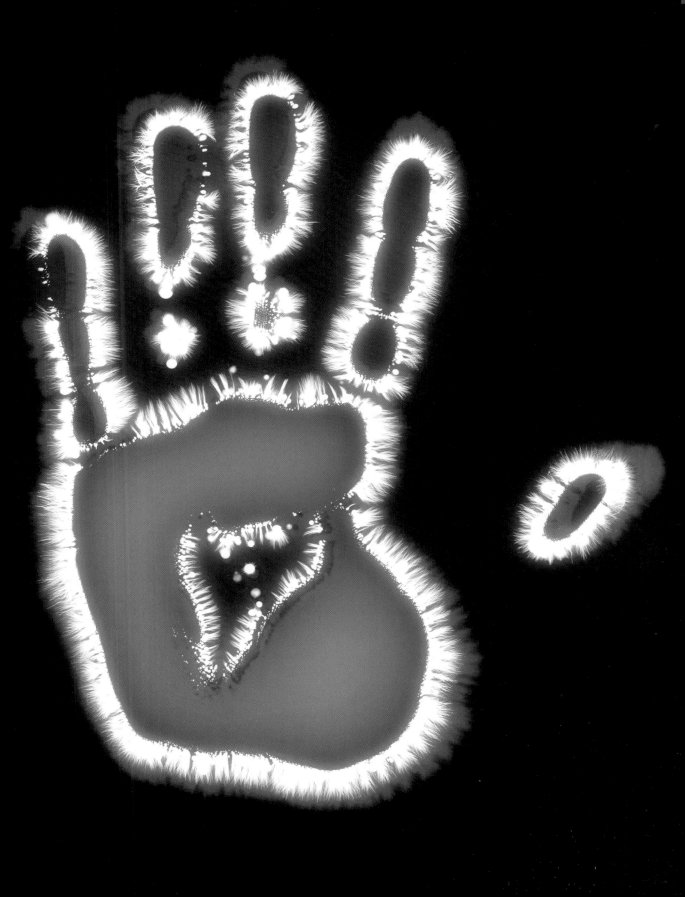

The seven energy bodies of the aura

Each energy body looks different and has its own function. Each one has an aura surrounding it that consists of electromagnetic radiation and gives us information, perhaps about emotional or mental well-being. We can learn how to "read" a person's aura and know what state (mental and physical) it is in. Also, each layer is associated with a particular chakra. For example, the first energy body is associated with the first chakra, and the second with the second chakra, and so on. The chakras are openings for energy to flow in to and out of the aura, as well as in to and out of the physical body. The fifth, sixth, and seventh energy bodies metabolize energies relating to the spiritual world, while the lower three energy bodies (first, second, and third) are associated with, and related to, the physical world.

The human aura

The aura surrounding each one of us is composed of seven energy bodies that merge and radiate outwards. The various colours of the aura can reveal important information about our physical, mental, and emotional well-being.

EXERCISE TO FEEL THE HUMAN AURA

This exercise helps you to tune in to your own energy field and make you feel more aware of your own aura (electromagnetic field). You will notice certain sensations flowing between the fingers and palms of your hands.

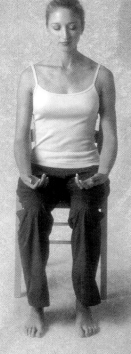

Step one

Sit on a chair or on a cushion on the floor; close your eyes for a while and start letting go of your shoulders with each out-breath (do this for three out-breaths). Simultaneously let go of any thoughts and tensions in the body.

Step two

Now hold your hands still in front of you, your palms facing each other, approximately 30 cm (12 in) apart. Relax and breathe in and out through your belly. Watch from inside, with closed eyes, the energy between your hands building up (do this for 2-5 minutes).

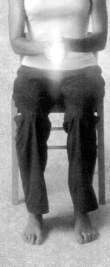

Step three

Now slowly move your hands towards each other, noticing the space between them. Become aware of the energy field between your hands. You will feel resistance.

Step four

Play with the space between your hands; coming closer, moving away. Notice sensations. You might get a feeling of tingling and pressure or a tickling sensation, like static electricity.

First energy body (Etheric)

The first energy body is the physical body, also known as the etheric body. Through the physical body we are able to exist on the material plane and gather experiences on this level. Our physical body, which works for us day and night, is a highly intelligent and complex system; all the organs function in harmony – for example, in order to digest food. Every seven years the body renews itself through rebuilding new cell tissue, and kidneys and liver are constantly working to detoxify the body. All physical functioning, physical sensations, feelings, and physical pain or pleasure belong to the first energy body.

STRUCTURE

The etheric body is the electromagnetic field of the physical body. It has the same structure as the physical body and includes all the anatomical parts and all the organs. The etheric body extends from one to five centimetres (one-quarter to two inches) beyond the physical body.

A healthy body is made up of fine lines of energy, similar to a delicate network of light. Some people can see "shadows" in the etheric layer that indicate disturbances of the physical body. These shadows change during the day and depend on whether the body is passive or active. The deeper and stronger a shadow, the more serious the physical illness. The stronger the physical body, the stronger the etheric layer: they are interdependent. We can learn about a person's physical health by reading his or her energy body.

VULNERABILITY AND STRENGTH

The healthier the physical body is, the stronger and more efficient the etheric layer is. The most important function of the first energy body is to protect the body from troublesome energy – for example, bacteria and viruses. A weak physical body with a weak etheric body is likely to be more vulnerable to disease. If the etheric body is strong it can easily resist bacteria and viruses: either they cannot penetrate the physical body or they are excreted immediately.

Clairvoyants and psychics can "see" the colours of the etheric layer, which pass from light blue to grey. An individual who is sensitive will be likely to have a similarly sensitive body, reflected in a bluish colour in the first layer. A person with a strong, tough body, will have a greyish colour in the first energy body.

The first energy body holds all the seven chakras, which resemble spinning wheels of light similar to the etheric layer. The chakras connect all the other energy bodies with the physical body and transmit information between each other. On the physical plane the chakras are connected with the endocrine glands (see the chart on p.30), which transmit subtle information from the other energy bodies into physical reactions. This is a complex system.

The first and second chakras direct energy to the physical body and without these functioning well life is not possible. Realizing the importance of the first energy body, we become more aware and more responsible about protecting and treating it with love and care, like a special friend.

To enhance your first energy body:
Self-relaxation exercise (see pp.14-15)
Dynamic Meditation (see pp.64-7)
Kundalini Meditation (see pp.74-5)
Vipassana Walking Meditation (see pp.96-7)
Guided relaxation and self-Reiki (see pp.108-9)

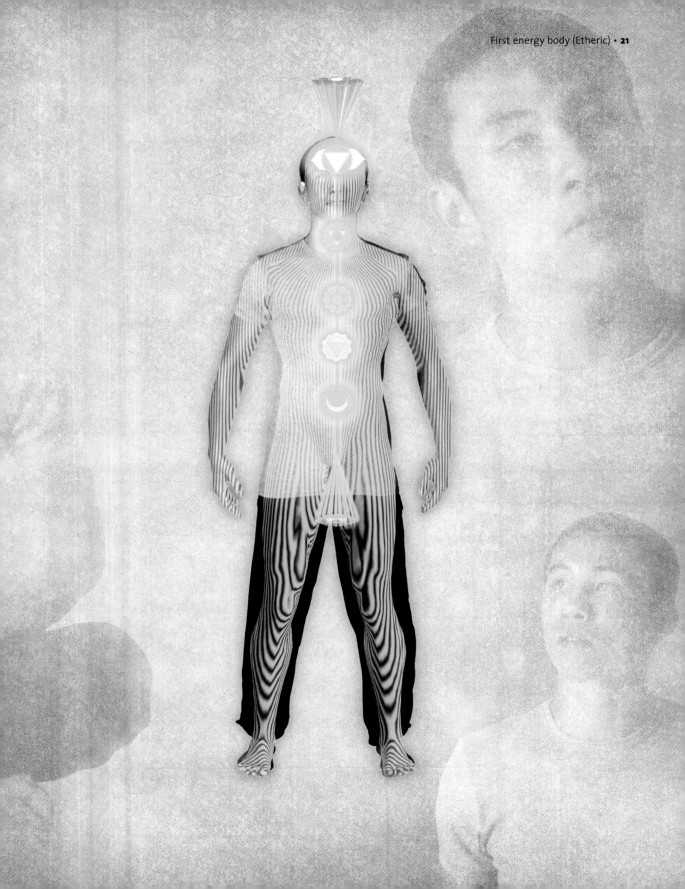

Second energy body (Emotional)

The next energy body after the etheric is the emotional body, which, with the second chakra, is connected with emotional aspects. Without this body we would not be able to feel emotion, as it registers feelings and becomes the vehicle through which we experience emotional life. All the emotional patterns that make up our personality are contained in it. The emotional body follows the outline of the physical body and the subtle energy vibration of this layer mirrors the emotional process that we are going through. Its structure is more fluid than the etheric body and to a clairvoyant it resembles clouds of multi-coloured light in fluid motion. This layer extends two and a half to eight centimetres (one to three inches) from the body.

ASSOCIATED COLOURS

The electromagnetic structure of this body depends on the refinement of the body itself. Clairvoyants "see" its colouring varying from bright to murky. All feelings are reflected in the second energy body and clairvoyants can distinguish the exact emotion a person is experiencing, seeing colours in the emotional body as the person changes from one feeling to another. For example, red indicates strong, forward-moving energy and it can also be interpreted as anger, while a soft red indicates tenderness, empathy, and joy. Our emotions often change quickly, reflected in the second body as confused energy. Clear and energized feelings such as love, excitement, joy, and anger produce bright, clear colours; feelings which create confusion produce dark, less distinct, hues.

These colours are accompanied by a special vibration and energy, which influences, for example, the atmosphere between individuals. Each feeling leaves an imprint in the emotional layer and a certain vibration, which radiates from the physical body and the aura. Imagine people meditating together with candles, flowers, and incense. They connect with their hearts and create a relaxing atmosphere, so that their emotional bodies can expand to release tension. This mutual energy is full of respect and love, creating a harmonious, nourishing vibration for the second body and our well-being.

CLEARING EMOTIONAL PATTERNS

The more we become aware of our negative emotional patterns and try to release them, the more refined and transparent our emotional layer becomes. The less we deal with negative emotional patterns the denser our second body and aura becomes. We might then feel angry, depressed, fearful, sad, and resentful. A dense emotional body can appear like a wall around the person. To clear and cleanse our emotional layer we need first to confront ourselves with fears and negative feelings. We need to have an honest desire to encounter emotional blockages and have the courage to face strong feelings.

Today there are different therapeutic methods for dealing with emotional patterns, allowing us to dig deeper into ourselves to look at the source of this negative pattern. This often goes back into childhood and if we have not become aware of it and been healed of it, our second energy body attracts the same situation repeatedly later on in our lives. If you know why you once created this emotional pattern – and it is clear that you do not need it any more – then you can let go of it. Slowly you create a distance from the pattern. Through dissolving old, stuck emotional patterns the second body becomes more refined and vibrates a positive energy.

To enhance your second energy body:
The Heart of Peacefulness (see p.46)
Mystic Rose Meditation (see p.47)
Dynamic Meditation (see pp.64-7)
Kundalini Meditation (see pp.74-5)
Guided relaxation and self-Reiki (see pp.108-9)

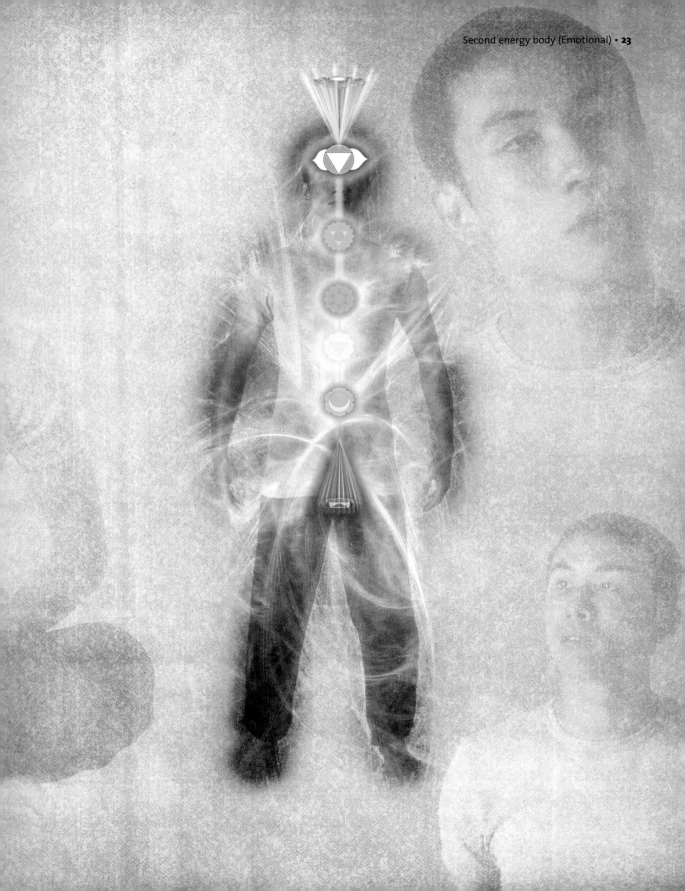

Third energy body (Mental)

This body extends beyond the emotional and consists of energies associated with our mental life, with thoughts and mental processes. The third energy body and third chakra are associated with linear thinking. Psychics "see" the colour of this body as a vivid yellow shining out from the head, shoulders, and the whole body. It expands and brightens when the person is mentally active, extending from eight to twenty centimetres (three to eight inches) from the body and even up to a few metres (yards), depending on the person's state of consciousness.

The mental layer holds our thought processes and mental creativity. Its high vibration produces constant thoughts and fantasies. Both the conscious and unconscious minds are active in the mental layer, so thoughts, desires, fantasies, fears, and hopes take place in this body. It is never resting, unless we are meditating.

THOUGHT FORMS

The third energy body holds thought forms or patterns. They appear to psychics and clairvoyants as spots of different shapes and brightnesses, carrying other colours, which radiate from the emotional layer. The current colour signifies the person's emotions associated with the thought form or pattern. By focusing on certain thoughts we enhance them. For example, thoughts and beliefs that were laid down in childhood can become so entrenched that they can dramatically influence our entire outlook on life. While we are growing up we learn certain rules and ways of surviving or fitting in to society. Some of these are helpful, maybe even vital, but some can become obstacles for individual and spiritual growth.

Over time we establish belief systems about ourselves, other people, and life in general, which can be negative or positive. If we carry negative thoughts or beliefs about ourselves, we limit ourselves and cannot live to our full potential.

For example, if you constantly think, "I am not good enough", "I can't do it", or "I am worthless". It is important to become aware of self-destructive and limiting beliefs and to decide where these feelings come from. Often we have to dig down deep into childhood memories. To purify the mental layer we need to free ourselves from negative thoughts and face our beliefs to uncover hidden thoughts.

A constantly nervous chattering mind forms a short cut in the mental body. The mind tends to think in terms of "good" and "bad", and "right" and "wrong", making instant judgements and forming rigid likes and dislikes. But when we become aware of and acknowledge a negative thought, it loses its power over us and can then be transformed into its positive form: "I am good enough", "I can do it", and "I am valuable". These positive thoughts purify the mental energy body. This creates a positive, more refined, energy vibration in the third body.

CREATIVE ABILITY

The ability to be creative is a part of the mental layer. Besides creating a better life on the practical plane – for example, by cooking a delicious meal – it is always a source of joy to create. If creativity flows freely in you, it feels like a source of vital energy that rejuvenates you. It is important to express creativity. You can do it simply by changing things in your home, such as hanging up a picture. Whatever you have always wanted to do and create, pay attention to it and translate it into action. This radiates a joy for life and connects you with a playful quality, which is part of the child in you.

To enhance your third energy body:

Nonsense Meditation (see pp.44-5)
Laughing Buddha Meditation (see pp.52-3)
No-mind Meditation (see p.93)
Reiki Mental Healing (see p.122)

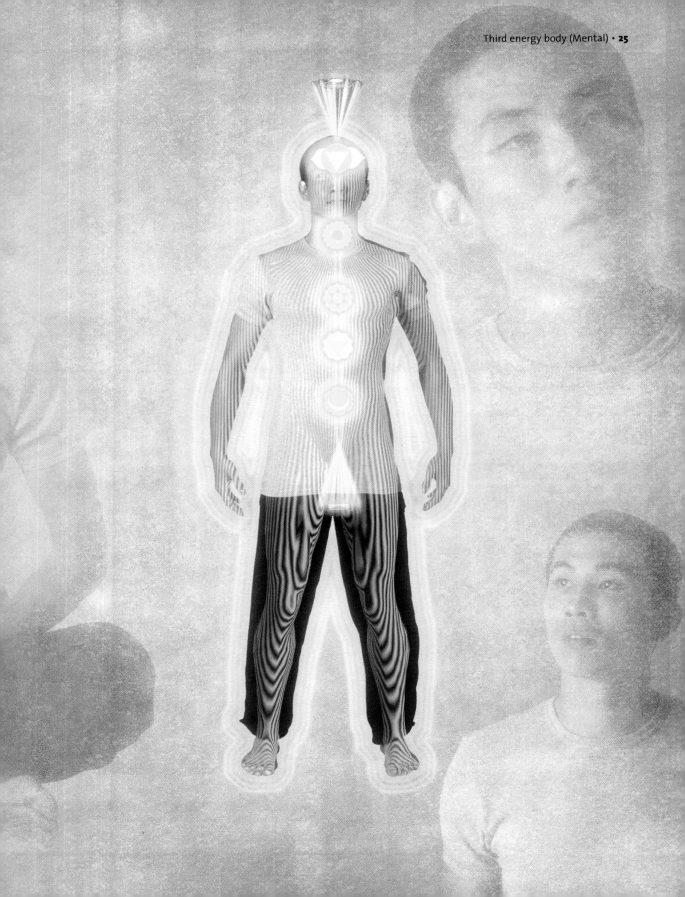

Fourth energy body (Astral)

The fourth energy body is associated with the heart (fourth) chakra. It is the vehicle through which we love others: family, friends, and people in general. The heart chakra is the energy centre that creates the energy of love.

To a clairvoyant the astral body consists of patches of different colours. It tends to have the same set of colours as the emotional body, but they are tinged with a pink cast. It expands to about fifteen to thirty centimetres (one half to one foot) from the body.

CONNECTING CORDS

The heart chakra of a loving person is full of rose light on the fourth energy body. When people form relationships with each other, they "grow" connecting "cords" out of the chakras. In a group of people or at a party, interaction takes place between people on the astral level. Patches of colour pass rapidly between individuals. Between potential couples, this is often a testing of the energy field to see if there is compatibility. It may be positive and enjoyable, but it can also be negative and uncomfortable.

To enhance your fourth energy body:

The Heart of Peacefulness (see p.46)
Emotional healing and balancing with Reiki (see pp.68-71)
Prayer Meditation (see p.79)
Reiki Distant Healing (see pp.124-5)

Fifth energy body (Spiritual)

The fifth energy body relates to the higher will, connected with the divine will ("Thy will be done"). The throat (fifth) chakra is associated with the power of the word, speaking, listening, and taking responsibility for our actions. The spiritual layer represents the divine spark in a human being and bears the individual's Higher Self, which is alert, full of light, and can see things clearly.

The Higher Self is free of feelings and thoughts, holding information about the plan in our lives and what we are supposed to do and learn. It has an overview of the person's life and takes decisions about their learning experiences. To be in touch with the Higher Self we need to first purify the first, second, third, and fourth energy bodies. The Higher Self cannot be in touch with us, and vice versa, when we are angry, sad, or in a chaotic state. But if we do our inner work and learn to meditate effectively, it is possible to contact the Higher Self and ask for its guidance, wisdom, and clarity (see Reiki Mental Healing, p.122).

The spiritual layer contains all the forms that exist on the physical plane. It resembles a photographic negative and is like a blueprint for the etheric body, which in turn is the blueprint for the physical body. The fifth energy body expands from about forty-five to sixty centimetres (one and a half to two feet) from the body. At the fifth level sound creates matter, so healing through sound is the most effective approach for this body.

To enhance your fifth energy body:
Stimulating chakra energy with sound (see pp.31-3)
Nadabrahma Meditations (see pp.88-9)
Mantra Meditations (see p.100)
Gayatri Mantra (see pp.116-17)

Sixth energy body (Cosmic)

The sixth energy body and sixth chakra are associated with celestial and divine love. It is a love that extends beyond human love. This love holds all life forms as precious manifestations of God. The cosmic layer extends about sixty to eighty-five centimetres (two to two and three-quarter feet) from the body. This is the level through which we experience divine ecstasy. We come to this state through meditation and inner work on ourselves. It is a state of being whereby we realize that there is no separation between ourselves and other living beings. We know our connection with all the Universe and we see the light and love in everything that exists. Our consciousness has risen until it has reached the sixth level, when we and God are a single continuum.

Some clairvoyants can "see" the cosmic layer. This layer appears similar to when you light a candle and the light radiates around it. The cosmic body emanates light all around with many rays of light.

To enhance your sixth energy body:

Golden Light Meditation (see p.92)
Full Moon Meditation (see pp.102-3)

Seventh energy body (Nirvanic)

The seventh energy body and crown (seventh) chakra are related to the higher mind, knowing, and integration of our spiritual life. The nirvanic layer extends from about seventy-five to a hundred and five centimetres (two and a half to three and a half feet) from the body. Raising our awareness to this layer creates a consciousness in us that melts with the divine consciousness so we are at one with existence: we come to the original source from which all existence originates and into which it returns.

The outer form is the egg shape of the aura, containing all the energy bodies related to the present incarnation an individual is going through. To a clairvoyant the seventh body looks like delicate strands of silvery light containing the aura's shape, in turn holding the form of the chakras and physical body. It thus creates a strong protective layer for the energy field.

To enhance your seventh energy body:
Sit silently in meditation
Vipassana Meditation (see pp.94-5)

The seven chakras

The seven chakras are specific vital energy centres in the body that influence different aspects of ourselves. They are energy vortices that govern our physical, emotional, mental, and spiritual well-being. The basic Reiki hand positions follow the seven main chakras and you can integrate the harmonization of the chakras into a single Reiki treatment (see pp.36-7).

OPENINGS FOR ENERGY

From a neuro-physiological perspective the chakras are represented as nerve plexuses from the spinal column and endocrine glands that connect with the internal organs. Each chakra opens to both the front and the back of the body. The front aspects of the chakras are concerned with the emotions and the ones at the rear with the person's will, but all seven chakras are openings for energy to flow into and out of the aura. Energy always has a specific manifestation or form, which we experience through the senses and through using our intuitive powers.

The chakras absorb universal energy (*ki, chi,* or *prana*), break it up into component parts, and then send it along energy lines called "nadis" to the nervous system, the endocrine glands, and the blood, to nourish the body.

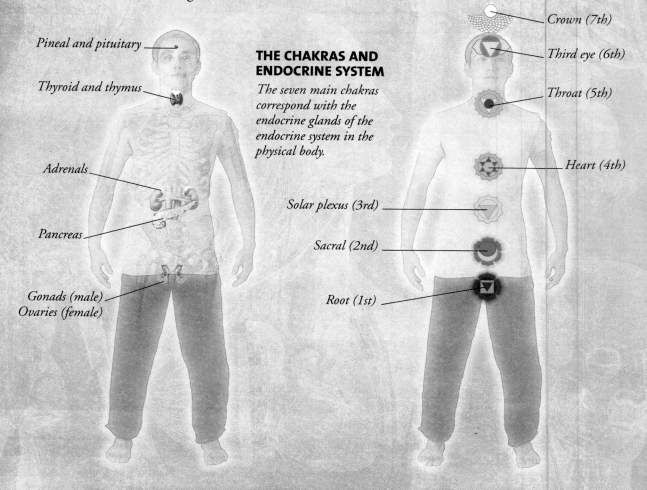

Pineal and pituitary

Thyroid and thymus

Adrenals

Pancreas

Gonads (male)
Ovaries (female)

THE CHAKRAS AND ENDOCRINE SYSTEM

The seven main chakras correspond with the endocrine glands of the endocrine system in the physical body.

Crown (7th)

Third eye (6th)

Throat (5th)

Heart (4th)

Solar plexus (3rd)

Sacral (2nd)

Root (1st)

DISTURBED BALANCE

Each chakra has its own energy vibration. If the vibratory frequency of a chakra is blocked or the chakra is rotating in the wrong direction, the balance in this chakra is disturbed. A person whose chakra energy is blocked or rotating in the wrong direction is easily manipulated and disturbed by others. Massage therapists report that they experience tightness and rigidity in their clients' bodies as a result of this dysfunction. When energy is held back from its natural flow – for example, when we suppress a feeling or if we stifle our actions because of fear – it will affect our etheric and physical body. The body then creates a protective barrier in the form and texture of our tissue.

Energy has to be constantly flowing through our system in order for us to remain in optimum health: inhibited energy flow can eventually contribute to ill health. Since the chakras serve to vitalize the body, it is important to open the chakras so that we increase our energy flow. Illness in the system is caused by an imbalance of energy, or a blockage, in the flow of energy. It affects our emotions and prevents us from living happily and contentedly.

STIMULATING CHAKRA ENERGY WITH SOUND

This energizing exercise stimulates the centres of the chakras. The crown chakra is not worked on. Try it whenever you need a little extra energy, either alone or with a partner. With a partner, stand facing each other, two or three metres (yards) apart, looking into each others' eyes. Do the exercise three times.

Step one

Stand with your feet a shoulder-width apart, slightly bending your knees. Take a deep breath, while stretching your arms upwards. Now make the sound: "Eeeeeeeee", as in "seek", while you are breathing out. This stimulates the third eye (sixth) chakra. If you are working with a partner, look into each others' eyes.

Step two

Take another deep breath and slowly open your arms, palms facing upwards, at shoulder level, chanting the sound "Aaaaay", as in "able". This activates the throat (fifth) chakra.

Step three

Take a deep breath, bringing the arms to a shoulder-width apart and bent at the elbows, palms facing up. Bend your arms and knees, and incline slightly from the waist. Now chant the vibration "Aaaaah", as in "art". This stimulates the heart centre (fourth chakra).

Step four

Taking another deep breath, bend forward from the waist. Bring your arms inwards, as if making a cradle, bending your knees. Now chant the vibration "Ohhhhhh", as in "show". This activates the solar plexus (third) chakra.

Step five

Take a deep breath again and squat down. Put your hands together in prayer attitude, or "namaste". If you are working on your own, place your thumbs together at the ridge between the eyes, above the nose. Make the sound "Oooooooo", as in "Do". This position stimulates the root (first) chakra and the sex centre (first and second chakras). Now repeat the whole exercise twice more.

Chart of the chakras

The chart below shows the positions and the various qualities of the seven main chakras of the body, as they are referred to in this book. They are a representation of the vital energy centres and different aspects of the human psyche: our physical, emotional, mental, and spiritual selves.

The chakras are rather like wheels or vortices, which spin, though they can become blocked or even spin in the wrong direction. The basic Reiki hand positions follow the locations of these seven main chakras, and they can make up a single Reiki treatment.

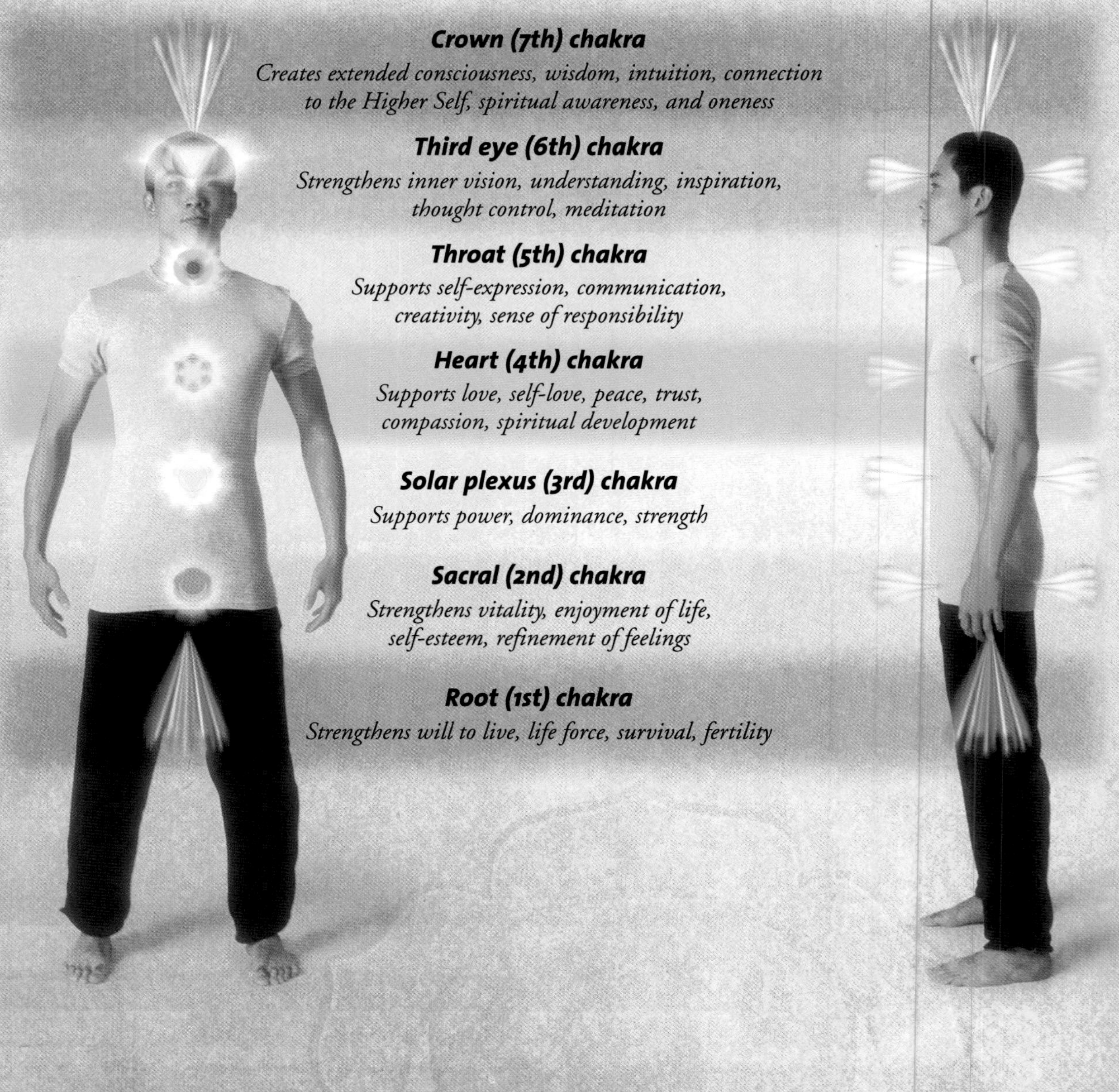

Crown (7th) chakra
Creates extended consciousness, wisdom, intuition, connection to the Higher Self, spiritual awareness, and oneness

Third eye (6th) chakra
Strengthens inner vision, understanding, inspiration, thought control, meditation

Throat (5th) chakra
Supports self-expression, communication, creativity, sense of responsibility

Heart (4th) chakra
Supports love, self-love, peace, trust, compassion, spiritual development

Solar plexus (3rd) chakra
Supports power, dominance, strength

Sacral (2nd) chakra
Strengthens vitality, enjoyment of life, self-esteem, refinement of feelings

Root (1st) chakra
Strengthens will to live, life force, survival, fertility

HOW BODY PARTS RELATE TO BEHAVIOUR

Our thoughts and emotions tend to shape our physical structure as well as the texture of our tissues in the body. Positive feelings keep the body supple and flexible, while suppressed emotions hold the energy back and create an energy block in the body. This can form a rigidity and *hardness in the body tissues. The body creates a protective barrier in the form and texture of our tissue. By relaxing the mind and contacting the inner self through Reiki and meditation combined, we can work on reducing rigidity in body tissue, wherever in the body it is most needed.*

Face
Expression of the various masks of personality; how we face the world

Nose
The heart, sense and smell, sexual response, self-recognition

Mouth
Survival, how we deal with security, the capacity to take in new ideas

Solar plexus
Expression of power and emotional control issues; the power wisdom centre

Abdomen
Seat of the emotions, contains deepest feelings, centre of sexuality, digestive system

Genitals
Relation to the root chakra, survival issues, fear of life

Knees
Expression of the fear of death, fear of change

Forehead
Intellectual expression

Eyes
Near-sightedness indicates a more withdrawn tendency; farsightedness indicates the more outward-looking windows of the soul

Jaw
Tension, indicating communication blockage; fear or ease of expression

Neck
Merging of thoughts and emotions, stiffness due to withheld statements

Chest
Relationship issues, heart and love emotions, respiration and circulation

Arms and hands
Extensions of the heart centre, expression of love and emotion

Thigh
Personal strength, trust in one's own abilities, fear of inadequate strength

Feet
Expression of groundedness, connection with reaching goals, fear of completion

Chakra balancing with Reiki

Vitalizing and balancing your own energy centres (chakras) with Reiki is very effective. As a rule there is often too much energy in the head and too little in the lower body. The crown (seventh) chakra does not need any additional energy, so you do not touch it in the course of balancing the chakras. Each chakra reflects an aspect of personal growth. If we have a block in the energy flow of our chakras, this may lead to an imbalance or a physical disorder. The locations of the chakras are shown on the chart (see pp.30 and 34), which describes the corresponding organs and characteristics of the chakras. With the help of Reiki you can harmonize an excess or shortage of energy in your chakras.

SELF-BALANCING THE CHAKRAS

This form of Reiki treatment is to help you vitalize and balance your chakras, to allow your energy to flow freely and keep you healthy.

Step one

Place one of your hands on your forehead (sixth chakra) and the other over the pubic bone (first chakra). This balances the energy of the head and the lower parts of the body. We often have too much energy in the head and too little in the lower abdomen. You will become more in touch with your sexual energy. Let your hands rest for about 5 minutes.

Step two

Lay one hand over your throat (fifth chakra) and the other on your belly (second chakra), below your navel. This balances the emotions and vitality with the area of self-expression and communication. You will feel more connected with your emotions and desires and be able to express them more easily in a creative way. Let your hands rest for about 5 minutes.

Step three

Lay one hand on the middle of the chest (fourth chakra) and the other on the solar plexus (third chakra). The heart stands for love and compassion and the solar plexus for your own strength and power. If these centres are balanced, the right decisions are made through love and understanding. Let your hands rest for about 5 minutes.

Step four

Place one hand on your belly in the navel area at the sacral (second) chakra and the other on the forehead at the third eye (sixth chakra). This position will relax you deeply and allow you to let go of thoughts and feelings. Let your hands rest for about 5 minutes.

Step five

After you have balanced all your chakras move your body gently, wiggle your toes and fingers, and stretch your whole body. Come back to normal consciousness.

Chapter two

The body and mind influence each other profoundly. Physical illness creates emotional stress, while emotional disturbances contribute to physical stress symptoms, such as insomnia.

Finding the **mind–body**

health connection

The mind has great power over the body, with the result that almost seventy per cent of diseases are mind-orientated, while only thirty per cent actually originate in the body. They may be expressed through the body, but their origin lies in the mind.

Since the 1930s, most traditional doctors have come to recognize the link between stress and illness and to realize that mind and emotions play a significant role. In the 1930s Dr Bach, an English physician, developed a method for using flower essences to harmonize conflicts in the mental–spiritual plane. Through his intuition and sensitivity he explored the healing effects of certain flowers. He was able to capture the energy frequencies of these flowers and conserve them in essence, developing thirty-eight remedies, which provide for every negative state of mind. By taking the right essence each mood can be redirected positively.

Today, holistic practitioners offer a wide range of therapies, such as Reiki, massage therapy, and acupuncture, to regain the patient's emotional health and well-being. Some holistic practices, such as hypnosis and colour-puncture, claim to detect diseases before they even occur. Colour-puncture uses Kirlian photography to diagnose the aura (see p.18) and show where a sickness is going to manifest – potentially, six months later.

STRESS REDUCTION

Many people suffer from stress and find it hard to relax. Happily, various techniques offer effective strategies for stress reduction including meditations, relaxation exercises, hypnosis, and physical exercise. Daily meditation is effective for helping people relax and with regular practice stress-related symptoms are less likely to manifest themselves. Active meditation also allows us to release tension in the body, mind, and emotions. We can tap in to a vast resource of creativity, knowledge, guidance, and inspiration from the Higher Self, which holds solutions to many of our problems. We can also use Reiki Mental Healing (see p.122).

Love

The heart knows how to love and when there is love there is also relaxation and mind–body health. The Japanese character for love lies behind the text on this page.

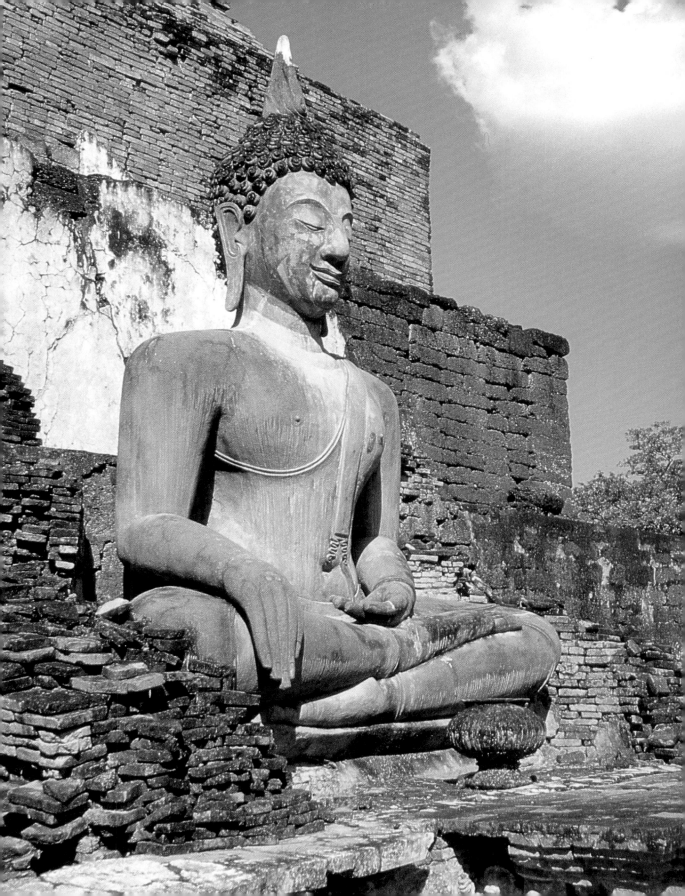

Tension

There are different types of stress that can affect us. Psychological stress is perhaps the most common. The individual's reaction to stress is based on their perception of some sort of threat to their well-being. This threat may be real or imagined, but it is always something that is either consciously or unconsciously perceived as threatening. Some people can cope better with stress than others. People who are good copers have fewer stress-related physical symptoms, a better-functioning immune system, and are less likely to fall ill.

EUSTRESS

In our rapidly changing society we come across many different demanding situations. To allow an individual to function as well as they can, stress researcher Hans Selye suggests that there is an optimal level of stress known as "eustress". He claims that a certain amount of stress is necessary to maintain good health, but if this level is exceeded, the person experiences "distress" and dysfunction. Some levels of stress trigger growth and help us to create strategies for dealing with new and demanding situations.

Most people acquire defence mechanisms and coping strategies for dealing with stress. For example, some people eat and drink too much in order to release their stress. Others build up physical symptoms or are prone to catching common infectious diseases such as coughs and colds, which shows that something is becoming too much for them. Others seem to flee into psychological illness to escape from environmental and psychological stresses.

WORRY

Much stress and tension is created through literally worrying ourselves sick. We fear that things will be different from the way we expect them to be or we anticipate the worst-case scenario of any given situation. We worry about the future and feel guilty about the past, especially when we feel responsible for the way things have turned out. We put demands and expectations on ourselves and on others. This is part of our human condition. We are constantly trying to be someone or something that we are not, and this creates pressure and tension in our lives. We are not satisfied with ourselves as we are and this longing can become physical. We may want to be better looking or to be better off, or better recognized for our achievements, or more emotional, more happy or contented, more powerful, more spiritual, or more liberated. The list goes on for ever. It does not really matter what it is that we want. Anything that we desire as something to be fulfilled in the future creates a tension between what we are now and what we long to become.

ACKNOWLEDGING FEARS

If we become aware of our fears or of any negative feelings, such as loneliness, unworthiness, or hopelessnesss, we need to acknowledge them before we can put them to one side. This process takes the "juice" out of any anxious or fearful feelings. We are back in the present moment and can start again from where we are now.

HUMAN IMAGINATION

Other life forms, such as fish or trees, cannot suffer from stress as we know it because they cannot imagine. Only humankind has the potential to imagine: we can project into the future and imagine what we are going to do tomorrow. This imagination is ours to use creatively and constructively, but it can also become destructive when we imagine ourselves as something that we are not.

QUICK REIKI STRESS-RELEASE TREATMENT

This quick treatment rejuvenates body, mind, and emotions. It is very effective after lunch or in late afternoon, when your energy may be depleted. Lie down or sit comfortably and relax. Cover your eyes with a blindfold or small beanbag (to create slight relaxing pressure on the eyeballs). Hold each hand position for between three and five minutes, for a total of 15 minutes.

Step one

As you breathe out, let go of any thoughts and tensions in the body with each out-breath. Repeat twice.

Step two

If you are lying down, cup the back of your head with your hands. If you are sitting, place one hand on your forehead and the other on the lower back of the head. This position calms the mind and emotions, and releases tension and headaches.

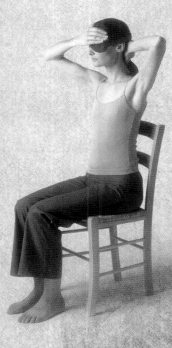

Step three

Now lay one hand on your navel and the other on your forehead. This position has a calming, centring effect. It treats the intestines and solar plexus.

Step four

Keep one hand on your navel and move the other to the middle of your chest. This position balances the energy from the heart centre (fourth chakra) and the sacral chakra (second chakra).

Relaxation

Only when we are at ease with ourselves and accept ourselves the way we are, can we let go of tension. To live in the present moment is ultimately to eliminate tension from our lives.

Relaxation happens when you stop living in the future or in the past, but live in the present instead. It is a state where your energy is not moving anywhere, but is simply there with you. There is no other moment, nothing to expect, nothing to ask for, nothing to want. Relaxation is a transformation of your energy. Normally your energy is motivated: moving towards a goal somewhere else. This dimension belongs to goal-oriented activity, whereby everything is a means to achieving something else. Somehow you have to achieve your goal; later you will relax. This kind of energy can dominate your life, continually changing into something else that you have to achieve. The goal is always on the horizon. You go on running, but the distance to the goal remains the same.

UNMOTIVATED ENERGY

However, there is another dimension to energy that is unmotivated. The goal is in the present, here and now. There is no other fulfillment than that of this moment. When the goal is not in the future there is nothing to be achieved. This moment is celebration, it is relaxation. And in this moment an overflow of energy, a response, or an unprepared action is taking place. We can do things and still remain relaxed. But how can we reach this state?

Relaxation techniques and meditation practices are the best tools for a preventative approach to health and well-being. Relaxation is complex and the best place to start is the body. Try doing everyday things in a more relaxed way. Slow down every process, every movement, to bring more consciousness into the physical body. If you try walking slowly, a new quality of awareness starts taking place.

Pay attention to your body and see whether you are carrying tension in your neck or shoulders, and then relax it consciously. Just go to that part and say to it lovingly, "Relax". The second step is to relax your mind. If you can relax your body, you will soon be able to relax your mind, too. The third step is to relax your heart. This realm of feelings and emotions is even more subtle. By now you are confident and can trust yourself. You have learned how to relax body and mind. The heart will follow automatically.

TALK TO YOUR BODY EXERCISE

This exercise will help you to get in touch with your body more easily and consciously release any tension. You acknowledge your body as a friend and understand it better. Do this exercise once or twice a day, for 5 to 10 minutes, or longer.

Step one

Lie down or sit in a relaxed position. Then close your eyes. Now go with your consciousness inside your body. Look for any tension in your body, from your toes to your head.

Step two

If you feel any tension anywhere, talk to that part of your body as if you are talking to a friend. Build up a dialogue between yourself and your body. Ask some questions: "How are you?", "Can I do anything for you?", "Can I release any tension or pain for you?" Then wait for an answer.

Step three

Thank your body for being so helpful and "there" for you, functioning endlessly and keeping you going.

Step four

Tell your body to relax and tell it that there is nothing to fear. Tell your body that you are there to take care of it. Slowly you will learn how to do this. Then your body will become relaxed.

Nonsense Meditation

This meditation acts out the continuous chattering of the mind, in a "nonsense" language. It relaxes the conscious mind deeply, so that body and heart can follow. This is also called the Gibberish Meditation. "Gibberish" comes from the Sufi mystic Jabbar, who spoke only gibberish. His message was, "Your mind is nothing but gibberish. Put it aside and you will have a taste of your own being." The mind always thinks in terms of words, so this nonsense language helps to break patterns of continual verbalization.

Use any nonsense words you like, or any "language" – for example, use "Chinese" if you don't know Chinese. Try the meditation initially for seven days, in the morning or evening, either alone or with others. Feel the effect of the meditation. After that, continue as and when you feel inclined.

STAGE ONE (15 minutes)
Step one

Sit or stand comfortably, feet a shoulder-width apart. Close your eyes, and begin to blurt out nonsense words or sounds. Sing, cry, shout, talk, whisper, or mumble.

Step two

Likewise, allow your body to express whatever it needs to express: jump, kick, lie down, or sit. Don't communicate with, or interrupt, anyone else. You can have your eyes open.

STAGE TWO *(15 minutes)*

Lie down on your front and feel your body sinking into the floor beneath you.

The Heart of Peacefulness

The heart is a natural source of peace. With this meditation you are simply coming back to your personal source of relaxation, which is always there. Being at peace contributes to good health. This technique helps you to become aware that your heart is filled with peace. When you have gone through these steps, relaxing the body, mind, and heart, you will be able to reach the innermost core of your being, which is the very centre of your existence. Then you will be able to relax this, too. This relaxation brings you joy, acceptance, trust, a deep letting-go, and surrendering.

You can do this meditation either sitting or lying down – for example, in bed on waking or just before you go to sleep. If you suffer from insomnia do the meditation at night and you will sleep deeply.

Step one

Sit up straight or lie down and relax. Close your eyes and let your breath flow naturally in and out. Now put your right hand in your left armpit and your left hand in your right armpit. Direct your whole attention towards your chest.

Step two

Allow a feeling of peace to rise from your heart. Just relax and focus on this feeling.

Step three

When you are centred here and relaxed, you will automatically contact your inner peace. The heart calms and transmits harmonic vibrations, which you experience as love and peace.

Remain for between 10 and 15 minutes in this position, enjoying this feeling.

The Mystic Rose

This technique purifies every layer of the body–mind and all the emotions. It is a deep cleansing of wounds and scars and can bring you in touch with your inner being. It is usually good to do in a group, unless you feel comfortable doing it alone. The short version takes one and a half hours and consists of three steps, each lasting half an hour. Do the meditation daily for a minimum of seven days and a maximum of twenty one. The long version, which lasts for twenty-one days, is done for three hours daily and preferably in a group. Do step one for seven days only. Then start with step two for the next seven days. Afterwards do step three for another seven days. During step three sit for forty-five minutes and then dance for twenty minutes. Then sit for forty-five minutes and dance again for twenty minutes. Finish with fifty minutes' sitting.

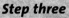

Step one

This part of the meditation removes all the things that stop you laughing. It creates a new space of relaxation within you.

Step one is just laughter. Laugh for no reason at all. At first you will have to do it deliberately, but the forced laughter will soon stimulate you to real laughter. After a while, it will become spontaneous. You may find that laughing causes tears to come. If you can, try to stick to the laughter for half an hour and then move on to step two.

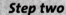

Step two

This step is crying. Just cry and start to feel any sadness, despair, or anxiety. So many tears have been suppressed. They are all there, and now is the time to let them come and to release any sad feelings you have.

Step three

The third step is sitting like the "watcher on the hill". Sit alert and comfortable for half an hour, watching your breath coming and going. Watch any thoughts that arise and let them pass by without judgement. (See also Vipassana Meditation, pp.94-5.)

The joy of life

Joy happens when your body, mind, and heart function all together. Joy is a quality of the heart. It arises out of an overflow of energy, love, peace, and harmony. It contains pleasure and happiness, yet is somehow more.

In the West we tend to live in our heads for most of the time and we use the left side of our brains predominantly. This is linked to our rational thinking processes. We seem to have forgotten the language of the heart. Only the heart knows how to relax, enjoy, and celebrate. Relaxation comes through the heart because the heart knows how to love and when there is love, there is relaxation. The heart is the most vital and fundamental part of us. The head is, in this sense, superficial. The important thing is to use both your head and your logical mind, but do not be used by them.

We may often get caught up in serious discussions and try to solve our own and other people's problems. If the mind tries to solve every single problem put to it, it will only produce anxiety, and can never be effective. As long as we stay in our heads, we will stay in our problems.

OPENING AND BALANCING THE HEART WITH REIKI

This treatment is very relaxing and opens the energy of the heart. It is very nourishing for the heart (fourth) chakra. Stay in each position for 3 to 5 minutes. Total treatment time is 15 to 25 minutes.

Step one

Sit in a chair or lie comfortably on the floor, with eyes closed. Place your hands loosely on your thighs. Take a deep breath and while breathing out make a little sigh with an "Ahhh" sound. Let go of your shoulders.

Step two

Put your right hand in your left armpit and your left hand in your right armpit. Focus attention on the chest area between your armpits and allow a feeling of calm, relaxation, and peace to come.

Step three

Continue sitting, or else lie on your back, and relax even more completely. Place your hands on your cheekbones, covering your eyes. Reiki energy affects the production of endorphins, the body's "happiness hormones". Make the sound "Yaa-hum" and allow the vibration of the sound to reach your heart. Do this for 3 to 5 minutes.

Step four

Place your hands on your chest or breasts, balancing male and female energies as well as the right and left sides of the body.

Step five

Place both hands on the abdomen on the navel, one hand above the other. Allow the Reiki energy to expand there. If you are lying down and you have lower back problems, put your feet up.

Reiki for enhancing well-being

Whenever you feel tense, tired, or worried it is worth taking the time to relax and make connection with yourself. Reiki can help you to relax your body and mind and to let go of tension more easily. To nourish yourself and feel better within yourself you can choose to do this treatment either sitting on a chair (as shown on these pages) or lying down. Remain in each hand position for about three to five minutes. The total time to allow for thes steps is a maximum of twenty-five minutes.

Step one

Sit in a chair or lie down comfortably. Relax your breathing and place your hands over your eyes, resting your palms on your cheekbones. This position balances the pituitary and pineal glands, which regulate hormones in the body and affect our emotional well-being.

Step two

Now place your hands on both sides of your head, above your ears, touching the temples. This position harmonizes both sides of the brain and has a relaxing and calming effect on the conscious mind. This improves clarity of thoughts, memory, enjoyment of life, and eases depression.

Step three

Now cup the back of your head with your hands. This position affects the unconscious mind and calms powerful emotions such as fear, worry, anxiety, and shock. It conveys a feeling of security and helps to calm and clarify thinking.

Step four

Lay your hands on the left and right side of your upper chest, fingers touching just below the collarbone. This position allows you to let go of negative feelings when you feel weak or depressed. It increases your capacity for love and enjoyment of life.

Step five

Place your hands at kidney height, fingers pointing towards the spine. This position treats the nervous system. It relaxes fears and shock, and enhances confidence. By releasing the middle back, we let go of the past and of stress and pain.

The laughing Buddha

There is a story in Japan about a laughing Buddha called Hotei. His entire teaching was laughter and nothing else. He would move from one village to another, stand in the middle of the market place and start laughing. That was his sermon and his ministry. His laughter was infectious. People could see his whole belly shaking with laughter and would start laughing, too. Then the laughter would spread, so that tidal waves of laughter would spread over the whole village. People used to wait for Hotei to come to the village because he brought such joy and celebration. He never said a single word. Laughter was his only message.

Laughter is like medicine, as it can change your very chemistry. It affects your brain waves and your thinking. Each and every good laugh releases tension in the body and reaches into the innermost part of your brain, to your heart. Nature has provided us with some very effective medicine, so that if you can laugh when you are ill you will regain your health sooner. Laughter brings energy from your inner resource to the surface. When this energy starts to flow for a few moments you enter a meditative state, where thoughts stop. You become possessed by the laughter. You cannot think and laugh simultaneously.

In some Zen monasteries the monks start and end their day with laughter. During the day they may feel laughter bubbling up because so many ridiculous, amusing things happen during an ordinary day. Laughter is helpful because it creates a distance between ourselves and our problems. Laughter can help you to become more detached and see the ridiculousness of life.

THE LAUGHING BUDDHA MEDITATION

This meditation will help you to laugh for no reason at all. If you can laugh early in the morning then laughter will come easily throughout the day and will lead to more laughter. Do this technique for between 5 and 10 minutes, with eyes open or closed.

When you wake in the morning, before you open your eyes, stretch and arch your whole body, like a cat.

After a minute or two, start to laugh. Simply lift the corners of your mouth and laugh, even if you do not feel like it. Soon forced laughter will stimulate the real thing and your laughter will become quite spontaneous. This will change the mood of your whole day.

Chapter three

Healing always comes from the heart and is a loving and accepting space we share with each other.

Intuition and awareness:

resonating together

Real healing takes place when both giver and receiver of a treatment resonate together. For this to happen we need to be tuned in on the same wavelength. For example, if you take two bells of the same tone and you hit one of them it will make the second one resonate and vibrate with the sound of the first. The same thing happens between two people. If the giver of a treatment is in a meditative state he is in touch with his "inner being", he is resting in his centre. From this place he can reach the "being" of the receiver and their two beings can meet and resonate together. Giving a treatment from this inner place allows us to recognize and embrace any illness, emotion, and hurts we are carrying. For any disease or hurt to be healed, it needs to be exposed, like a wound to the sun, in order for the person to become whole and healthy again.

REIKI FROM A RELAXED SPACE

Practising meditation will relax you more and help you to get in touch with your own centre. To give a Reiki treatment from this relaxed and meditative space inside allows your ability to heal to emerge and come alive. This will deepen your

Reiki. In turn, Reiki will bring balance and harmony to your body and enhance well-being.

REIKI GUIDELINES

Reiki is a non-intrusive, peaceful, and loving way to transmit healing energy. Healing happens when it is sent from the heart. Before you give Reiki, spend some quiet time in contemplation and meditation to centre yourself and create a loving atmosphere that encourages relaxation for both giver and receiver. As the giver, stay in a receptive state and remind yourself, before offering treatment, that you are being used as a channel for healing. Show gratitude for this in your own way. During the treatment stay alert and present. Be available for the energy to travel through you. You do not need to activate or consciously send energy. Just be present and enjoy the moment. If it feels right, after the treatment, discuss anything that either of you noticed.

Understanding

Exercising intuition and cultivating awareness leads along the path of understanding. The Japanese character for understanding lies behind the text on this page.

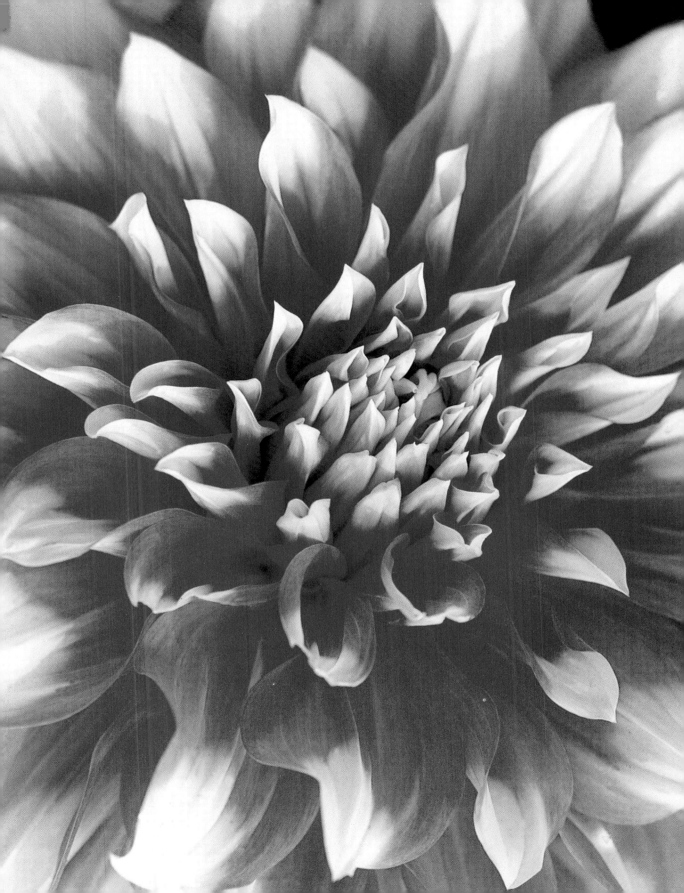

Basic Reiki hand positions

Before you start to practise intuitive Reiki, the next six pages give a reminder of the basic Reiki hand positions used in a full-body treatment and as they are taught in the First Degree Reiki training. Remain in one hand position for between three and five minutes. You will be able to sense when a part of the body has received enough Reiki. In some areas you may experience heat or cold. Here, let your hands rest until you sense that the energy flow has normalized.

Head position one
Lay your hands to the right and left of the nose, covering forehead, eyes, and cheeks.

Head position two
Lay your hands on the temples, with fingertips touching the cheekbones, the palms following the shape of the head.

Head position three

Lay your hands over the ears. This position affects the whole body.

Head position four

Cup the back of the head, with the fingertips over the medulla oblongata *between the head and the neck.*

Head position five

Lay your hands at either side and above the front of the throat – do not touch the throat directly.

Front position one

Lay one hand across the thymus gland, below the collarbone, the other at right angles to the first, on the breastbone, in the middle of the chest (together the hands form a "T").

Front position three

Lay one hand on the lower ribs on the left side, below the chest, the other directly below it at waist level.

Front position two

Lay one hand on the lower ribs on the right side, below the chest; the other directly below it, at waist level.

Front position four

Lay one hand above, the other below, the navel.

Front position five ("V" position)

If the receiver is a man, place your hands in the groin area, without touching the male organ. If the receiver is a woman, lay both hands over the pubic bone.

Back position one

Lay both hands on the shoulders, one hand to the left and the other to the right of the spine, hands facing the same direction.

Back position two
Lay your hands on the shoulder blades.

Back position three
Lay your hands on the lower ribs, above the kidneys.

Back position five (A), or "T" position
Lay one hand across the sacrum, the other at right angles to the first, over the coccyx, to form a "T".

Back position four
If the receiver has a long back, move your hands to the lower part of the back (at hip level).

Back position five (B), or "V" position

Lay the fingertips of one hand directly on the coccyx and lay the other hand so that it forms a "V" with the first.

Knee hollow position

Cover the hollows of the knees with your hands.

Sole position (A)

Lay your hands on the soles of the feet, ideally with fingertips covering the toes.

Sole position (B)

Rest the palms of your hands on the toes and point your fingertips towards the heels.

Meditation guidelines

You can try different types of meditation. One type is active, another is passive, or silent. Yet another uses visualization and contemplation. The active techniques usually contain phases of physical activity and cartharsis to unload any tension in the physical and emotional body.

The Indian mystic Osho devised contemporary meditation methods that are used by people all over the world. Many of his techniques are introduced in this book – for example, Dynamic Meditation (see pp.64-7). The techniques are particularly important for Westerners. This is because in the Western world the predominant lifestyle tends to be active. People seem to live on the periphery of their being and identify strongly with such values as prestige, wealth, power, and physical looks. These values lie outside the individual.

Western society is male-orientated and the overall energy is outgoing. The slogan "Go for it!" sums up the feeling and many people lose contact with their "divine" selves. Inner resources and values, such as trust, compassion, love, self-love, and real understanding between people seem to struggle for existence.

We may accumulate possessions and aspire to ever-higher standards of living, but we remain frustrated at still not finding happiness and contentment. We cannot find a meaning to life, and we don't know who we are or why we are here. We can only find the answers to these questions by ourselves, inside ourselves. We need to learn how to go in to ourselves and meditation techniques are the right tools for doing this. To look inside yourself starts you on a journey and opens up your inner world, so that you can come to know yourself.

MALE AND FEMALE ASPECTS

To practise meditation you need to be passive, non-doing; this is female energy. Each person carries male and female aspects inside and to be in touch with both parts, in balance, is ideal. The three essentials in meditation, which must be present in every technique, are: be watchful of your body, as it slowly relaxes; be in a relaxed state of mind, without controlling it, without forcing your concentration; and watch whatever is going on with a relaxed awareness, without judging and without evaluating.

Meditation is a function of being happy.
Meditation follows a happy man like a shadow.
Wherever he goes, whatsoever he is doing,
he is meditative.

Osho, The Everyday Meditator

UNITY BETWEEN PEOPLE

In the silence we stop feeling separate from one another. We go beyond our personalities and develop compassion and understanding. Also, we see things from a higher perspective. If people meditate together, the effect of each meditation is to create unity between people. We become one and the painful feeling of being separate dissolves. Meditative qualities are vital for the spiritual development of the whole of humanity.

During meditation try to remain playful and patient and keep an experimental approach uppermost. Do not look for instant results; instead, explore and be relaxed. If you find that a particular meditation suits you better than others, do it for a minimum of seven days and a maximum of two months. Then evaluate the effects it has on you and continue, or try a new meditation technique. When you start meditation, you need to make an effort just to prepare yourself and release tension in the body. Choose active meditation techniques initially, then later on choose silent methods – for example, Vipassana Meditation(see pp.94-5), where you just sit in meditation.

Dynamic Meditation

Dynamic Meditation is for releasing emotions and increasing your general awareness. When doing this meditation you feel more alive, vital, and vibrant with energy. This technique connects you with your root (first) chakra and sexual centre. It consists of five phases: breathing, exploding, jumping, freezing, and celebrating. While you are doing this meditation you remain in your centre. This is only possible because of the first three steps of the meditation, which prepare you for the stillness of the last step. The last stage is to dance in celebration and enjoyment.

It is best to do this meditation early in the morning, on an empty stomach, and to keep your eyes closed for the duration. The process lasts for one hour. Special music is available to accompany the meditation (see p.139).

Step one: Breathing (10 minutes)

Breathe rapidly in and out through your nose, concentrating on the exhalation. The breath should move deeply into the lungs, and the chest expands with each inhalation. Do this as rapidly as you can, without tensing your body, and keeping your neck and shoulders relaxed. Continue until you literally "become" the breathing. Allow your breathing to become spontaneous, rather than steady or predictable. Once your energy is moving, it will begin to make your body move in an expressive way. Allow these movements to happen; don't suppress them. Feel your energy building up. Don't let go yet and don't slow down.

Step two: Exploding (10 minutes)

*Let go of your body and express whatever you need
to express. "Explode" and let your body take over.
You may want to scream, cry, jump,
kick, shout, shake, dance, laugh,
and sing. Let go of everything
within you that needs to be
thrown out. Go utterly mad.
Keep your whole body moving,
hold nothing back. Don't let your
mind interfere with what is
happening. Be total! In the
beginning a little acting may
help to get you started.*

Step three: Jumping (10 minutes)

Raise your arms as high as you can, straight over your head, without locking your elbows and keeping your shoulders and neck relaxed. Jump up and down shouting, "Hoo, hoo, hoo" as deeply as you can, so that it comes from the bottom of your belly. Each time land on the soles of your feet (making sure your heels touch the ground), let the sound hammer deep into your sexual centre. Exhaust yourself totally.

Step four: Freezing (15 minutes)

STOP moving completely. Freeze in whatever position you find yourself. Don't feel self-conscious and don't rearrange your body in any way. Even a cough or a slight movement will dissipate the energy flow and the effort will be dispersed. Now be a witness to everything that is happening to you.

Step five: Celebrating (15 minutes)

Now celebrate and rejoice with music and dance. Express your joy, whatever is there. Feel very alive and carry your aliveness with you through the rest of the day. You can keep your eyes closed or open.

Emotional healing and balancing

When we worry and feel emotionally upset, tension and energy seem to gather around the head. To balance this energy and to bring it down to other parts of the body, start by treating the head with Reiki. All the following hand positions balance powerful emotions such as fear, confusion, shock, and worry. Try the following positions on a receiver and ask them to stay in each position for about five minutes. The whole treatment takes forty to sixty minutes.

Step one

Place your hands over the eyes, resting palms on the cheekbones or eye sockets. This position balances the hormones as it affects the pineal and pituitary glands. It also helps to reduce emotional stress and facilitates meditation.

Step two

Lay the hands on both sides of the head, above the ears, touching the temples. This position harmonizes the two sides of the brain. It helps to ease stress and depression, and calms the mind.

Step three

Place your hands over the ears. This position gives a comforting and secure feeling, and has a relaxing effect on the whole body.

Step four

Cup your hands under the head. Treating the back of the head makes the receiver feel secure. This position relieves fears and depression and calms the mind and emotions.

Step five

We strengthen the heart and increase the capacity for love and enjoyment of life by using the "T" position or laying the hands on the middle of the chest for self-treatment. A feeling of general weakness and depression can be transformed.

Step six

Place one hand on the lower abdomen, just below the navel, and the other on the forehead. This position relaxes the receiver deeply and helps him/her to let go of thoughts and feelings.

Step seven

To release further emotions and tensions lay your hands flat along the insides of the thighs, between the upper legs with your fingertips pointing in opposite directions. In this position the receiver can let go of deep-seated fears, often held in the stomach area.

Step eight

Now place your hands on both knees. We often hold tension and fear of death in our knees. By giving Reiki we can release this fear.

Step nine

Ask the receiver to turn over. Now place your hands on the lower ribs, above the kidneys. Treating the middle back helps the receiver to let go of the past, stress, and pain.

Step ten

Now lay your hands on the soles of the feet, ideally with fingertips covering the toes. Alternatively, rest the soft part of your palms on the toes and point your fingertips towards the heels. This is good for strengthening the root (first) chakra, and it grounds all their chakras, plus all other areas of the body.

Step eleven

Place one hand on the lower back and the other on the medulla oblongata *between the head and the neck. This position gives a feeling of security and being taken care of.*

Step twelve

Smooth the aura from head to toe twice, then draw an energy line from the base of the spine up over the head.
   Take a few moments to come back to normal consciousness, and allow time for your receiver to come back, too. Stretch your body and wiggle fingers and toes. You will feel more connected with yourself; more nourished and balanced.

Intuitive Reiki

This "expanded" form of Reiki treatment allows you, as the giver, to connect with your intuition. To be available to your own inspiration and wisdom, to put your hands where they "want" to go, and to trust this process is an exciting experience. Reiki opens up your intuition and trust. You allow your hands to move wherever they are drawn. This often indicates an area where there is tension, a lack of energy, an imbalance, or a pain that needs to be released.

MEDITATION FOR INTUITIVE REIKI

The receiver lies down on a blanket on the floor or on a treatment table. Keep another blanket nearby. Treatment time is between 30 and 40 minutes. Do not play music between steps one and six.

Step one

Connect with your centre and empty yourself of thoughts, tensions, and feelings. With each of your out-breaths, let go a little more and breathe out any tension.

Step two

Tune in from your heart. With both hands, gently touch the head of the receiver above the ears. Close your eyes. Now be receptive and open yourself to receive any information or message from your receiver. A "message" is where you feel a need for the receiver's body to be touched in a certain place. This can seem to be a lack of energy, an imbalance, or tension in the body that needs to be released. Messages can include a visual picture, sounds, or words that tell you something about the emotional well-being of the receiver.

Step three

Use your intuition and wait until you feel like continuing.

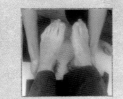

Step four

Now go to the receiver's feet. Hold the heels in each hand. Close your eyes. Take a deep breath or two and connect with your own centre. Relax and open yourself to accept any information from the receiver's body. Get a clear picture of where the person wants to be touched. You may notice tingling sensations in your hands.

Step five

Sit on one side of the body at the level of the receiver's waist. With eyes closed tune in and connect with the receiver. Hold one of her/his hands and wait for the contact between you to build. Wait until the impulse to move on comes.

Step six

Now place your hands on the body, wherever you feel drawn. Use your inspiration and intuition to know where the body needs healing and continue with Reiki treatment. The treatment can last for 30 minutes, or longer. If you wish, play relaxing music. At the end of the treatment hold the receiver's feet for a short time, cover her/him with a blanket, and allow time for returning to normal consciousness.

Kundalini Meditation

This meditation helps you to free your body of any tension by being in stillness with yourself. It consists of four stages of fifteen minutes each: shaking, dancing, witnessing, and being still.

It is best to do this meditation in the afternoon or early evening. Meditation time is one hour. Special music is available to accompany this meditation (see p.139).

Step one: shaking (15 minutes)

With eyes closed, stand silently, be loose, and let your body shake. When your body starts trembling a little, help it along. Welcome it, but don't force it. Feel the energies moving slowly up from your feet. Let go everywhere and "become" the shaking.

Step two: dancing (15 minutes)

Keeping your eyes closed, dance in any way you like, and let your whole body move as it wants to.

Step three: witnessing (15 minutes)

Keeping your eyes closed, be still, sitting or standing. Start witnessing whatever is happening inside and out. If you are sitting, place your open hands loosely on the upper legs, with palms up, or rest them in your lap in front of you.

Waiting is meditation.
Waiting with full awareness.
And then it comes…,
it cleanses you, it purifies you,
it transforms you.

Osho, The Orange Book

Step four: being still (15 minutes)

Keeping your eyes closed, lie down on your back, and be still.

Releasing worries with Reiki

To stop worrying and relax yourself or your receiver, use some of the basic Reiki head positions (see pp.56-61). They help to let go of negative emotions and balance the function of the pituitary and pineal glands, which themselves govern hormonal balance. There is also an increase in the secretion of endorphins, the body's so-called "happiness hormones".

You can use this treatment on yourself or on a receiver. Hold each position for about five minutes, or longer.

Step one

Place your hands over the receiver's eyes, palms resting lightly on the cheekbones or eye sockets. This position balances the pituitary and pineal glands. Use it for treating exhaustion and stress. Relaxing the eyes has the effect of relaxing the whole body.

Step two

Lay the hands on the left and right side of the receiver's head, above the ears, touching the temples. This position harmonizes the two sides of the brain, helping to ease stress and depression, and calming the mind.

Step three

Cup your hands beneath the receiver's head. Use this position for calming powerful emotions, such as fear, shock, and for tension and headaches. It is good for depression and brings clarity to the mind. By treating the back of the head we convey a sense of security.

Step four

Now continue to give Reiki to the chest area. For women (self-treatment): place your hands directly over your breasts. This balances the left and right sides of the body and harmonizes the male and female sides. For men (self-treatment): place your hands next to each other, covering the whole chest. Rest in your heart centre (fourth chakra) and connect with your feeling side. When treating a female receiver it is very important to ask for feedback and permission to treat in this position.

Step five

Now place your hands over the solar plexus area, below the breasts and above the waist. This will give you strength, enjoyment of life, and trust.

Step six

If you are treating a receiver, ask her/him to turn over. Give Reiki to the kidneys and adrenals by placing your hands in the middle of the back. As you relax and relieve pressure on the adrenal glands, the production of adrenaline slows.

Step seven

When you are treating a receiver, continue by treating the upper shoulders. Lay your hands on the outside of the shoulders, pointing your fingertips towards the arms. This releases emotional stress and tension, and helps circulation of the blood in the arms and hands.

Step eight

Smooth the receiver's aura twice and allow time to come back to normal consciousness. Then draw an energy line from the base of the spine up to and over the head.

If the receiver has a headache, is fearful or confused, try Rescue Remedy to help relieve stress. Mix six drops in a glass of water, to be drunk throughout the day, or while the period of difficulty lasts.

Prayer Meditation

This meditation allows you to merge with the energy surrounding you. You feel as if you are flowing with the energies of earth and heaven, in which Yin and Yang, male and female, energies mix. This merging with energy is prayer; it changes you. It is best to do this meditation at night, in a darkened room, and then go to sleep immediately afterwards.

If you do it in the morning, allow time for fifteen minutes' rest immediately afterwards.

The whole meditation takes about twenty to thirty minutes. Special music is available to accompany this meditation (see p.139).

Step one

Kneel down and raise both your hands; your palms face upwards and your head is raised. Feel cosmic energy flowing into you; fill yourself with the energy of the sky. Be like a leaf in the breeze, trembling, while the energy flows down your arms. Let your whole body vibrate with energy.

Step two

When you are completely filled, usually after 2 to 3 minutes, bend down and let your forehead touch the ground, palms down. You become a vehicle, allowing the energy of the sky to unite with the energy of the earth.

Repeat the first and second steps at least seven times; more if possible. Any fewer and you will feel restless and unable to sleep. Each of the chakras will become unblocked.

Step three

Go to sleep in this state of prayer. This energy will surround you for the whole of the night and it will continue to work within you. By morning you will feel vital and refreshed.

Advanced chakra balancing with Reiki

Using Reiki to balance the energy centres (chakras) is very effective. As the basic Reiki positions follow the seven main chakras, numbered one to seven, you can integrate the harmonization of the chakras into a single Reiki treatment. You can also treat the energy centres separately. The process usually takes fifteen to twenty minutes.

Each chakra reflects an aspect of personal growth. If the chakra energy flow is blocked, this may lead to an imbalance and to a mental, spiritual, or physical disorder. With the help of Reiki you can harmonize, or balance out, an

excess or shortage of energy in your chakras.

As a rule there is often too much energy in the head and too little in the lower body. The crown (seventh) chakra does not need any additional energy, so do not touch it in the course of this treatment. Allow the hands to rest on the two chakras that require balancing until you can feel the same energy in both. You may feel a temperature difference between the two points, ranging from warm to cold. If this is the case, wait until you feel both hands becoming the same temperature.

The treatment lasts for forty minutes.

Step one: Smoothing the aura

Let the receiver lie down on his/her back. Arms should be relaxed on either side. Smooth the receiver's aura from head to toe, using smooth, curving movements, starting at the head and working down to the feet. Do this three times. It has a relaxing effect on the receiver and prepares for treatment.

Step two: Root (first) and third eye (sixth)

Lay one hand on the root chakra and the other on the third eye chakra and remain there until you can sense the same amount of energy flowing in both centres. When treating a woman you can touch the pubic bone, but when treating a man hold the hand a short distance above the pubic area.

Step three: Sacral (second) and throat (fifth)

Lay one hand on the sacral chakra and the other just over the throat chakra, but without actually touching the throat. Rest there until you sense balanced energy between both centres.

Step four: Solar plexus (third) and heart (fourth)

Lay one hand on the solar plexus chakra and the other on the heart chakra. Rest there until you sense balanced energy between both centres.

Step five

You can now deepen the healing with emotional balancing. Place one hand on the lower abdomen just below the navel and the other on the forehead. After a couple of minutes move your hand clockwise in extreme slow motion on the lower abdomen a few times. This creates deep relaxation for the receiver and helps him/her to let go of thoughts, feelings, and any tension in the body.

Step six

To release further emotions and tensions lay your hands flat on the insides of each thigh, between the upper legs (fingertips pointing in opposite directions). This will help the receiver to let go of fears, which are often held in the stomach or belly area.

Step seven

Ground the chakras and all areas of the body by giving Reiki to the feet. Rest the soft parts of the palms of your hands on the toes and point your fingertips toward the heels. Or lay your hands on the soles of the feet, ideally with fingertips covering toes. This strengthens the root chakra.

Step eight

At the end of the treatment smooth the aura again from head to toe twice, then draw an energy line from the pubic bone up over the head.

The chakra breathing technique

This meditation can help you to become aware of and experience the energy in each of the seven chakras (see also pp.30 and 34).

Use deep, rapid breathing and body movement to open and bring awareness and vitality to the chakras. While breathing it is helpful to shake your body, stretch, tilt, or rotate your pelvis. You can move your hands however you want, but let your feet stay in one spot. Allow your feet, knees,

and hips to become like springs, so that the movement becomes continuous and effortless.

The best time to do this meditation is in the morning, on an empty stomach, or during the late afternoon, before your evening meal. The meditation lasts for one hour, during which your eyes remain closed. Special accompanying music is available (see p.139).

Step one

Stand with feet a shoulder-width apart. Let your body relax. Your eyes are closed and your mouth is open. Breathe deeply and rapidly, in and out in a second, into the root (first) chakra. Pay attention to the pelvic area, where the first chakra is located. Breathe in a rhythm that feels comfortable and allows you to become aware of the feelings and sensations of the chakra. Breathe into the first chakra for about a minute and a half.

Step two

Then move and breathe into the sacral (second) chakra. Don't force your breathing, but breathe in a rhythm that feels comfortable. Become aware of the feelings and sensations of this chakra and breathe into it for about a minute and a half. As you pass through the chakras, your breathing becomes more rapid and more gentle.

Step three

Move this deep, rapid breathing up into the the solar plexus (third) chakra. Your breathing becomes progressively more rapid and more gentle.

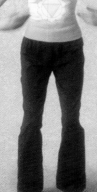

Step four

Now move into the heart (fourth) chakra, still maintaining deep, rapid breathing, becoming increasingly rapid and gentle.

Step six

Move into the third eye (sixth) chakra.

Step seven

Move into the crown (seventh) chakra, by now taking twice as many breaths as in the first chakra. Allow awareness to turn and fall through each chakra, letting your breath slow. Let the energy flow from crown to root chakra. This takes about 2 minutes.

Step five

Move into the throat (fifth) chakra.

Step eight

Stand silently then move and stretch. Go back to the first chakra and continue breathing up the chakras. Repeat this three times over 45 minutes.

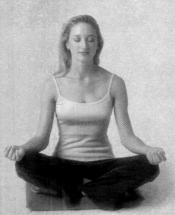

Step nine

After the third sequence of upward and downward breathing, sit with closed eyes in stillness for 15 minutes. Become aware and watch whatever is happening inside.

Reiki for colds and flu

Having a cold or flu is often a sign that something has become too much for us, that our body system is suffering from stress. We need a break to spend some time with ourselves; the body is demanding our attention. Reiki is the ideal tool to give energy and support to ourselves in these circumstances. We can soothe our aching symptoms and often speed up the healing process.

Treat yourself with Reiki every morning and evening for about thirty minutes. Do these positions while you are either lying in bed or in a sitting position.

Step one

Start by treating your head using head positions one, two, three, and four (see also pp.56-7). These positions ease inflammation in your sinuses and inner ear, but all head positions are a great support when you experience pressure and aches in the head.

Head position one

Place your hands over your eyes, resting your palms on the cheekbones.

Head position two

Place your hands on both sides of your head, above your ears, touching the temples.

Head position three

Place your hands on both sides of your head, covering the ears.

Head position four

Cup the back of your head in both hands.

Step two

Now lay your hands on either side of the throat. This strengthens the lymphatic system by treating the lymph nodes and it helps a sore throat.

Step three

This position stimulates the thymus gland. Use it for strengthening the immune system and lymphatic system. Give Reiki here for about 10 minutes.

Place your hands on the front of the body, below the collarbone, fingertips touching in the middle, on the upper breastbone.

At the same time try using some Bach Flower Remedies (see p.38). A mixture of walnut, olive, crab apple, clematis, hornbeam, and mustard strengthens and supports your inner cleansing and healing. Mix three drops of each remedy in a glass of water and drink it throughout the day, for a period of 5 to 10 days.

Nadabrahma Meditation

This humming meditation has a powerful calming and healing effect. It is an old Tibetan technique and was originally practised by Tibetan monks in the early morning hours. It can be carried out at any time of the day, alone or with others. If you practise it in the early morning it is advisable to follow it with a pause of fifteen minutes before starting your day's activities.

The meditation consists of three stages and lasts for an hour. The first two stages are accompanied by relaxing, special meditative music (see p.139).

STAGE ONE (30 minutes)

Sit in a relaxed position, with eyes and mouth closed. Start to hum, so that you can hear yourself easily and let the vibration spread through your whole body. Imagine that your body is hollow inside, like a bamboo, and is completely filled by the vibration of your humming. Make a humming noise when you breathe out.

STAGE TWO (15 minutes)
Two steps of 7½ minutes each.

Step one

Hold both your hands in front of your body, palms upwards. Move your hands in a circular movement away from your body. Your hands move forwards, then separate in two large circles to right and left. Do this so slowly that it seems as if your arms are hardly moving.

Step two

After 7½ minutes, turn your hands over so that the palms are downwards. Now move your hands in the opposite direction. Your hands meet near the navel and then separate again on both sides, tracing large semicircles. Feel how you are receiving energy. If you want to, gently move your body, too.

STAGE THREE (15 minutes)
Sit or lie on your back and remain absolutely still and silent.

Nadabrahma Meditation (couples)

This is a variation of the exercise for couples, ideally of the opposite sex, so that male and female energies can interact, but same-sex pairs can enjoy it and gain benefit from it, too. Humming together will help the energies to

meet, merge, and unite. Light the room with four small candles and burn a favourite incense. If possible, reserve this incense just for burning during this particular meditation.

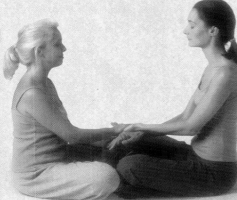

STAGE ONE

Sit facing your partner, holding each other's crossed hands. If you want to you can be naked and covered with a sheet. Close your eyes and hum together for 30 minutes. Feel the energies melting into each other.

STAGE TWO
Step one

Hold your hands in front of your navel, palms upwards, moving your hands away from the body in two symmetrical circles, to left and right. Feel how you are giving out energy.

Step two

After 7 ½ minutes, turn your palms downwards. Now do the opposite movement. Hold your hands in front of your navel and then separate them on either side, tracing semicircles inwards. Feel how you are receiving energy.

STAGE THREE

Sit or lie on your back and remain absolutely still and silent, each with one leg over and one under the other's. Hold your partner's legs.

Reiki to refresh your energy

Giving yourself Reiki healing is always rejuvenating and it recharges your batteries. If you treat yourself on a daily basis the refreshing effect may be even more noticeable. You will feel generally healthier, your immune system will be stronger, and you will look and feel more vibrant. Carry out this treatment either sitting or lying down. Hold each hand position for approximately three to five minutes and for a total of thirty minutes (maximum).

Step one

Get comfortable in a sitting or lying position. With each out-breath feel your body sinking deeper into the floor beneath you.

Step two

Now lay your hands over your eyes, palms resting on your cheekbones. This position balances the pituitary and pineal glands, which regulate hormones and affect relaxation.

Step three

Now place your hands on both sides of your head, above your ears, touching the temples. This position helps to ease stress, calm excessive mental activity, and soothe the mind. It also alleviates headaches.

Step four

Now cup the back of your head. This position conveys a sense of security, relieves fears and depression, and calms the mind and emotions.

Step five

Lay your hands on the left and right sides of your upper chest, fingers touching, just below the collarbone. This position strengthens the immune system, regulates heart and blood pressure, and stimulates the lymph circulation. It transforms general weakness and negative emotions.

Step six

Lay your hands on your solar plexus, over the lower rib cage and above the waist. This position restores energy, promotes relaxation, and reduces fear and frustration.

Step seven

Place your hands around the waist at kidney level, fingers pointing towards the spine. This position strengthens the kidneys, adrenal glands, and nerves. It helps to detoxify the body, promotes relaxation, and reinforces self-esteem and confidence.

Golden Light Meditation

The following technique works with male and female energies. The visualization of golden light helps to cleanse the body and to fill it with creativity; this is male energy. The visualization lof darkness entering makes you receptive, calms you, and gives you rest; this is female energy.

Do this meditation twice a day. The best time is early in the morning, just before you get out of bed. When you are coming out of sleep you are very receptive, operating less in the mind. Start the technique the moment you feel you are fully awake. The second-best time to do it is when you are going to sleep, at night.

If you fall asleep while doing the meditation, do not worry: the impact will remain in the subconscious and will go on working overnight.

Carrying out this meditation, which takes twenty minutes, over a three-month period will let the energy gather normally at the sex centre, or root (first) and sacral (second) chakra, and then flow upwards. Special music is available to accompany this technique (see p.139).

Step one

Lie on your back with your eyes closed. While breathing in, visualize light entering your head and going into your body. Let it enter through the top of the head, the crown chakra. Visualize that the sun or moon has risen just close to your head and allow golden light to pour into your head. Imagine you are hollow, like a bamboo, and the golden light is going deep down into your body, down to your feet, and out through your toes.

Step two

When you breathe out, visualize darkness entering through your toes. Imagine a great dark river or the darkness of the night entering your body through your toes, flowing up through the body and going out through the head. Breathe slowly, so that you have time to visualize. Stay with this image. To recap: when you inhale, light (male energy) is coming in; when you exhale, darkness (female energy) is entering the body.

No-mind Meditation

For this meditation use any language that you do not speak or know (see also Nonsense Meditation, pp.44-5). Simply allow whatever comes into your head to express itself in words and sounds that have no particular meaning for you. This technique enables you to get rid of your thoughts without suppressing them.

Try this meditation for seven days in the first instance, in the morning or evening, either alone or in a group. Feel the effect of the meditation. After that, continue with the meditation if you want to.

Step one *(45 minutes)*

Sit or stand comfortably, close your eyes and begin to say nonsense words or sounds: sing, cry, shout, talk, whisper, or mumble. The mind always thinks in words, so this nonsense language helps to break up the pattern of continual verbalization. Likewise allow your body to express whatever needs to be expressed: jump, kick, lie, or sit down. Do not interact or interfere with other meditators.

Step two *(45 minutes)*

Sit comfortably with closed eyes and witness everything that is happening inside you.

Step three *(5 minutes)*

At the end of the meditation, relax your body and let it fall backwards, just like a bag of rice, and relax for a few minutes, without moving at all.

Vipassana Meditation

Vipassana is a Buddhist meditation developed by Gautama Buddha 2,500 years ago. Many thousands of disciples became enlightened through this technique of witnessing breath, actions, body, thoughts, emotions, and environment, without reacting. It is an invitation to get to know yourself and make friends with yourself. You become detached from what you are witnessing; there are no results, nothing special is supposed to happen, and nothing is expected.

One way of doing this meditation is to become aware of your body, mind, emotions, and moods. Another is to become aware of your breathing. For women it is easier to watch the breath by noticing the rise and fall of the belly. For men it may be easier to become aware of the breath going in and out through the nostrils, producing a certain coolness. While watching your breath other things will distract you: thoughts, feelings, judgements, body sensations, and pain. Whenever possible, go back to watching the breath. It is the process of watching that is significant, not what you are watching. Do not become involved with what comes up; just let it float away.

Meditate at a regular, pre-selected time and place for forty to sixty minutes. Although this is the ideal time, just try twenty minutes initially and slowly increase the time as you get used to sitting still. Sit on the floor cross-legged or in a chair. Your spine and head should be straight and it is best not to lean against anything. You can do this meditation alone or with others, with eyes closed and breathing normally. Sit as still as you can, moving only if necessary. If you do move, notice why and how you are moving.

Sitting for forty-five minutes can be followed by fifteen minutes of Walking Meditation (see pp.96-7).

VIPASSANA TECHNIQUE FOR BEGINNERS

In the beginning, just sit for 20 to 30 minutes. Then slowly increase the sitting time as you get more used to sitting still.

STAGE ONE

Sit in a relaxed position on the floor or on a chair. Hold your spine straight and relax your shoulders. Now place one hand on your navel. Feel the rise and fall of your belly as your breath passes in and out. For the next 5 minutes keep your hand there and say silently "In" while breathing in. Then say "Out" while breathing out. This helps your mind focus on the breath. If you focus on your nostrils, do the same when you feel the breath actually touching them.

STAGE TWO

Rest your hands loosely on your upper legs. Now watch and catch hold of your thoughts by "naming" them. This means putting a name to a thought when it arises. For example, say "food" if you think of food, or "movie" if you think of a movie, or "dog" if you think of your dog, and so on. Find just one word for a thought and say it twice silently. Do this for 5 to 10 minutes. Then let go of this, too.

STAGE THREE

Now pay attention to whatever is happening. This includes thoughts, feelings, body sensations, judgements, pain, any impressions from the outside world. When you remember, go back to watching your breath.

VIPASSANA FOR ADVANCED MEDITATORS

This technique is also known as "Watching the Gap in the Breath". Gautama Buddha tried this method and among Buddhists it is known as Anapanasati Yoga.

Instructions

First become aware of breath coming in. Now move in tune with consciousness of your breath. When the breath goes in, you go in. Then go with the breath while breathing out, fully conscious. Before the breath turns in or out, there is a moment when you are not breathing: the gap in the breath. It is not easy to catch this gap, but if you go on practising breath consciousness, suddenly you will come to it. As your awareness becomes deep and intense, you will feel the gap, the moment when the breath is neither going out nor coming in, but has stopped completely. This is "the beneficence".

Vipassana Walking Meditation

Normally, when we walk the mind becomes very active; we do not even notice what the body is doing. Only when we are interrupted do we become aware of it and are thrown into the present. Walking and becoming aware of each movement is a meditation; relieving tension and calming the mind. This technique is based on the awareness of the feet touching the ground. You can walk in a circle or a straight line of ten to fifteen steps back and forth, indoors or outdoors.

Instructions (15 minutes)

Walk slowly, with your awareness focused on your feet as they touch the ground. Keep your eyes lowered to the ground, so that you can see only a few steps ahead. If you like, place your hands on your heart centre. While walking pay attention to the contact of each foot as it touches the ground. As you walk in slow motion you can say, "Right" when the right foot touches the ground, and say, "Left" when the left foot touches the ground.

If other things arise, notice what else takes your attention, and then return to your feet.

General Awareness Meditation

Anything can become your object for witnessing. Any action, any daily routine, such as eating, washing-up, cleaning the house, talking, jogging, dancing, or reading, can become a meditation.

Be aware of the movements and sensations of your body, while you are walking, eating, or taking a shower. Just be alert. Meditation can enrich the quality of everyday life.

Nataraj Dance Meditation

This meditation allows you to get lost in dance. You melt and merge with it. Forget the dancer, the centre of the ego, and become the dance. The division between dance and dancer disappears: then it becomes meditation. If you get totally involved in the dance, the dancing is no longer an act, it is a *doing*. You are not watching yourself and how you are dancing. Instead, you are allowing the dance to flow in its own way. You are just playing with your own life energy. This is a happening and a celebration. Special music is available to accompany this (see p.139).

STAGE ONE *(45 minutes)*

With eyes closed dance as if possessed. Involve yourself totally in the dance. Dance so deeply that you forget you are dancing. Do not watch or control your movements; instead, let the dance flow in its own way. Begin to feel that you are the dance.

STAGE TWO *(20 minutes)*

Keeping your eyes closed, lie down on the floor immediately. Be still and silent.

STAGE THREE (*5 minutes*)

Dance in celebration and enjoy yourself.
Be playful. Your eyes can be open or closed.

A really meditative person
is playful;
life is fun for him,
life is a leela, a play.
He enjoys it tremendously,
He is not serious, he is relaxed.

Osho, The Orange Book

Mantra Meditations

Mantras are Sanskrit syllables, words, or phrases designed to heal and bring a higher state of consciousness. They are ancient and their origin is often unknown. Sounds and mantras are used in meditation to activate the energy in the upper chakras to reach a higher level of vibration and awareness. When you intone the sound "AUM" you will become harmonious with it. It is as if the sound is entering your body, contacting every part of you. You feel rejuvenated and energized.

THE AUM MEDITATION

You can do this meditation alone or in a circle, standing or sitting, with friends. Do it as long as you like, though between 10 and 30 minutes is ideal.

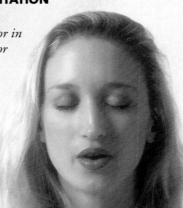

Step one

Intone the sound "AUM" aloud. Then gradually feel filled by it. Let the sound vibrate through your whole body, through your mind, your whole nervous system. Intone it and feel that every cell of your body is filled with it. Tune yourself in to the sound. The more you feel deep harmony between yourself and the sound, the more you will feel yourself filled with a subtle sweetness.

Step two

When you begin to feel harmonious with it, you can intone "AUM" inside silently, or whisper it. Your whole body dances with it. It is bathing in the sound, as though every pore of your skin is being cleansed. Make the sound more slowly and more subtly, letting your awareness grow.

HUMMING MEDITATION TECHNIQUE

Close your mouth lightly and hum a low and deep sound, keeping the same note all the way through. The vibration of the sound affects the heart centre (fourth chakra) harmoniously. This will bring peace to your whole being. Do it for 10 to 20 minutes, once or twice a day. (See also Nadabrahma Meditations, pp.88-9.)

The art of energy returning to you

In our daily lives we give out energy all the time, without noticing it. Much of it travels in and out through the eyes, when we are looking and trying to absorb information. This means that we are continuously giving out energy, but without it returning to us. As we have learnt to be extroverts, we give energy out and we lose it. This technique helps you to let the energy flow back to you, and is very valuable.

Step one

Look at your reflection in the mirror. Then let the image look back. Start feeling that you are being looked at by the reflection in the mirror, so the energy can flow back to you. In the beginning it will be subtle, but you will notice a change in the energy. Something of immense power starts entering you and energy moves back into you. You feel very much alive.

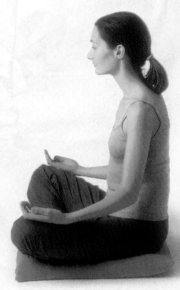

Step two

Look at a rose for a few minutes. Then allow it to look at you. You will be amazed at how the energy can change and how much the flower can give to you. You become introverted and energy flows back to you. Practise with any other object in nature, such as a tree, the moon, the stars.

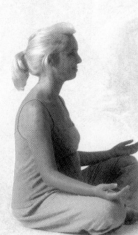

Step three

Look into the eyes of a friend or a beloved. First look at her or him and then start feeling that they are returning the energy back to you. Notice the change in the energy. Carrying this out simultaneously, you will both be rejuvenated and revitalized.

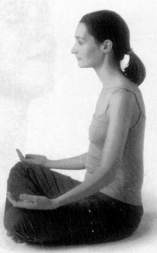

Full Moon Meditation

This meditation can fill you with the serenity and calm of the moon, making you feel thoroughly contented and relaxed. The mystical qualities the moon emanates enter and possess you, allowing you to draw on its energy. Start doing this technique three nights before the full moon and then do it again on the night of the full moon itself. You can also talk to the moon, ask questions, and then perhaps receive answers. Be as expressive and uninhibited as you like.

Step one

Go outside, under open sky, look at the moon and start swaying.

Step two

Slowly start allowing the energy of the moon to enter you. Feel as if you are becoming possessed by it. Continue moving gently. Continue swaying from side to side and making expressive arm movements.

Step three

Look at the moon, relax, and ask it to do whatever it wants with you.

Step four

If you feel like singing and dancing, then do so. Allow whatever wants to happen to happen.

As the moon becomes fuller you will feel more energy. On full moon night spend an hour outside, swaying, singing, and dancing. Allow the moon to possess you.

Mastery of moods

We often suffer from our own mood swings. Until we move to our own centre and relax, knowing "this too will pass", we will not be at one with ourselves. This story gives deeper insight into the ever-changing events in our lives.

A king who felt frustrated with life asked a Sufi mystic for a ring. This ring could make him joyful when he was unhappy, but if he was happy he could look at it and feel sad. What he was really asking for was mastery of his own moods.

The Sufi mystic had a ring which had a carving under the precious stone. When he gave the ring to the king he said, "There is one condition to having this ring. You should look at it only when everything is lost. Otherwise you will miss the message." The king obeyed. His country was threatened and he was fleeing for his life. The king ran, but he came to an abyss. At this moment he opened the ring, and read the message. It said, "This, too, will pass".

Whether you are happy or unhappy, remember 'This, too, will pass'. This key allows you to become master of your moods instead of their victim.

Osho

MASTERY OF MOODS EXERCISE

Do this exercise 5 minutes before you start working. It will refresh you with new energy.

Step one

Sit silently and relax. Become aware of your breathing.

Step two

Allow your dark mood to leave you with each out-breath. Do this consciously for about 5 minutes.

Meditation for plane travel

In a plane gravitation is lessened and you can easily and effortlessly achieve a meditation. It is also a very good way of passing the time. This exercise allows you to enter a feeling of vastness and space that is inside you as well as all around you. Feel that you are surrounded by clouds, stars, and vast space. Now get in touch with this feeling of vastness.

Step One

For a few moments imagine that your body is becoming bigger and is filling the whole airplane.

Step Two

You are growing bigger and bigger – bigger than the airplane. And the airplane is now inside you.

Step Three

Now imagine and feel that you have expanded into the whole sky. The clouds and stars are moving inside you. You are boundless – unlimited.

Rising in love together

Unless a relationship between a man and a woman is very conscious, it is bound to be problematic. There is a deep attraction between the couple, which we call "falling in love". The same opposition that creates the attraction between the two can transform into conflict.

Men and women have different attitudes and approaches and very often they fail to understand each other. A man's way of looking at the world is different from a woman's. If both partners are conscious of this fact, then this is a meeting of opposites and a great opportunity to understand the other's point of view and absorb it. To deepen your love you will need to meditate, and as your meditation develops, your love rises.

Meditation gives your love eyes and understanding. To sit together with your partner and meditate connects you with the innermost core of the other person. Through meditation you will receive the insight to understanding your opposite. You will also receive the qualities of awareness, silence, patience in listening, and capacity for understanding each other. (See also Nadabrahma Meditation for couples, p.89.)

EXERCISE ALONE
Step one

Sit alone. Remember the conflict, issue, or problem with your partner. Now imagine that you are him/her and try to put yourself in that position. If you are a woman, try to see as a man sees and if you are a man, try to see as a woman sees.

Step two

Speak out loud to yourself:
"I am (name of partner)."
"I am wearing a …."
"My job is …."
"This is my situation (describe the conflict from your partner's point of view)."
"I am feeling …."
"My partner thinks that I am … and this makes me feel …."
And so on, continuing the talk as you need to.

Step three

Come back to yourself and see whether you have any insights.

EXERCISE TOGETHER

You can do this playful exercise at any time, any place. Decide on the length of time, perhaps starting with 5 or 10 minutes.

First swap roles: you are your partner and you play your partner's role. Use his/her words and phrases, act out appropriate physical attitudes and gestures, and anything that is typical of him/her. At the same time, your partner does the same with you. Next, notice how you felt while you were playing each other. Notice how it affects you. Share insights with each other.

Exercise using cushions

Put a cushion in front of you to symbolically represent your partner and sit on one yourself. Imagine your relationship is no longer an ordinary relationship: you have both become fellow travellers on a spiritual path. A man and a woman are two parts of the same whole and understanding each other is the key to dissolving conflicts.

Step one
Start talking about your problem with your partner–cushion and then switch roles and "be" your partner by sitting on the cushion opposite.

Step two
Speak out loud, "I am (partner's name)". Continue as in the second part of exercising together – see opposite.

You can switch roles any time you need to. Just be aware that you sit on the partner–cushion when you are talking as if you were your partner and sit on your own cushion when you are talking as "you". During your talk you can ask your partner questions, but wait and sit on the other cushion to answer them. Whenever you change cushions, give yourself time to adjust to the new role.

NB: *Be prepared for feelings to surface. You can always ask a friend or counsellor to be present or support you.*

Guided relaxation and self-Reiki

You can use this exercise to help you to guide yourself into a healing relaxation. You can make a recording of the instructions first, but leave three minutes' silence or play an interval of relaxing music after each step. Alternatively, just do one step after the other and play the music continuously throughout the whole treatment. Suitable music: Gregorian chants, didgeridoo playing, overtone singing, or mantra singing.

Step one

Lie down comfortably and relax, eyes closed. Cover yourself with a blanket. Take a few deep breaths and let go of any thoughts and tensions in the body while you are breathing out. Feel your body sinking deeper into the floor with each out-breath.

Step two

Place your hands anywhere on your body where it feels right, or where you need some support. Allow Reiki energy to flow into your body. Now sink even deeper inside yourself and relax (play music for 2-3 minutes).

Step three

Slowly move your hands to another part of your body and give Reiki there (play music for 3 minutes).

Step four

Move your attention to the inside of your body and explore it. If you come across any dark corners, notice them. Now send some light to these dark areas. Let the light enter from the top of your crown (seventh) chakra and allow it to flow into your body. Also let the light emanate from your hands into your body.

Step five

Now sink even deeper inside yourself. Let yourself be touched by something higher than you, higher than your personality: a divine force, a divine energy. Going even deeper into an unknown space inside yourself, the healing that is needed for you can happen now. Allow another 10 minutes, with or without music, for relaxation and healing to take place.

Chapter four

Remembering who we truly are is a key to self-healing.
We are beings of light embodied in a physical form,
at one with the Universe and God.

Healing and spiritual

growth: divine connection

Once we begin to understand that we are beings of light embodied in a physical body and that we are at one with the Universe, God, and the true selves of others, our consciousness begins to change. We must be responsible for our actions and become more aware of their consequences. Recently, people are realizing that thoughts and emotions affect health. Emotional blockages can manifest in the physical body and affect the function of the chakras and our immune system.

To give and receive love is an important human need. Expressing love towards ourselves and others is significant for health and well-being, so we must learn to be more loving and giving. But we need to love ourselves first before we can truly love others. To express love is perhaps one of the most important lessons to learn.

We need to find the real reasons for illnesses. In this new millennium we encounter a new era in human consciousness. Healers and psychics talk of a shift of human consciousness taking place, due to higher vibrational frequencies of love on earth. We are making the transition into a new dimension, where our hearts open and we begin to remember our divine connection. So we need to forgive ourselves and others, transform fear and give up attachment, frustration, and negativity, and understand oneness. Old, unconscious patterns of separation, manifested in emotional energy mindsets, denial, likes and dislikes, are fading. We are facing a situation where we must choose to cooperate or suffer. We are moving together towards a new collective consciousness of peace, love, and harmony.

Reiki is a powerful healing art that supports the individual. Giving and receiving Reiki means sharing gifts, our love, with each other. It diminishes the feeling of being alone. By using Reiki tools we raise the vibrational frequency of the body; our intuition becomes stronger and we establish a deeper level of communication with our Higher Self. Through Reiki and meditation we develop greater awareness of ourselves and finally reach a clear perspective about "who we truly are": a divine being of light.

HARMONY
Reiki brings harmony to individuals so they can share a deep love and understanding with others. The Japanese character for harmony lies behind the text on this page.

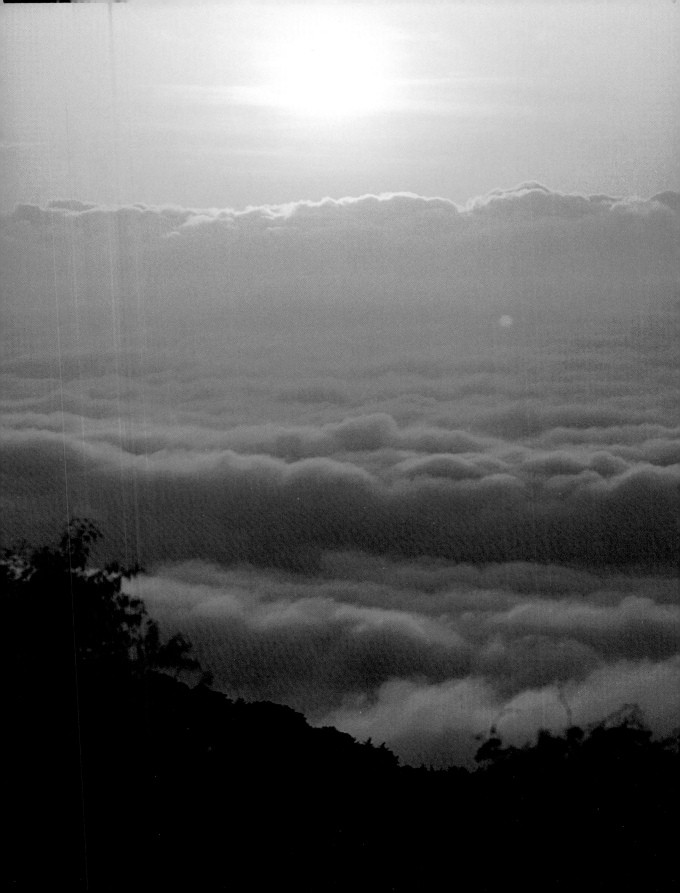

The Reiki principles

Dr Mikao Usui (1864–1926) is the discoverer of Reiki. He established the spiritual precepts for life, as we have been told, more than a hundred years ago and they still carry as profound a meaning for us today as they did in his own time.

Up until now, Reiki students in the West have been taught that Dr Usui worked in the Beggars' Quarter of Kyoto, Japan. As he realized that the beggars he treated free of charge did not feel appreciation for their healing, he was very disappointed. He had hoped that they would reintegrate into society and start to live a normal life. Now, the story goes, he became aware of how important it is that a person really wants to change his or her life and therefore needs to participate in their own healing process. He also saw that, by giving away healing, he had actually strengthened the beggar pattern in them rather than weakened it.

He understood that people must give something back in return for their healing, in order to maintain healthy balance in their lives. This is sometimes called an "energy exchange". Usui left the Beggars' Quarter and searched for those who really longed to be healed. Those who were true seekers he gave the Principles of Reiki, so that they could heal themselves.

Lately, however, research has revealed that Usui was not a Christian Minister in a university in Kyoto, nor did he work in the Beggars' Quarter. Instead, he was a Buddhist and he spent his entire life seeking enlightenment. Reiki became a path for him to achieve this. Usui is supposed to have healed the victims of the great Kanto earthquake, which devastated Tokyo in 1923 and he was honoured for his good deeds by Emperor Meiji of Japan.

In his lifetime Usui founded the Usui Reiki Ryoho Gakkai (Usui Reiki Healing Method Society) in Tokyo and became its first president. Shortly after his death the Japanese organization built a memorial for him at the Saihoji temple in the suburbs of Tokyo. The inscription on Usui's memorial talks about his life, his purpose in life, about the Reiki method and the five principles. The inscription mentions that the principles are invented by Emperor Meiji and that Usui took them on board. He recommended that the principles should be used in daily life and that they should be followed as guidelines, to be contemplated in the heart of each person, to heal their lives and thoughts.

These principles appear to be very simple. However, it is important to be aware that they should be recognized for their far deeper purpose. It is well worth looking at them in depth, to understand their inner meaning.

1. "JUST FOR TODAY, I WILL LET GO OF ANGER"

"Just for today – thou shalt not anger".
This guideline indicates the importance of becoming more conscious of our feelings. We all carry anger within us and often we do not know what the real source of it is. Anger can be triggered by a minor incident and the real reason for it may be unconscious. For example, your young child breaking a cup may cause you to feel an explosion of anger building up for the child, when deep down you are really angry with your partner, who does not give you enough attention.

Whatever the cause of our emotions, we truly need to look at each situation as though we are looking in a mirror, at the reflection created by us. Those who stimulate our anger may not necessarily be the main cause of it. Beneath each feeling of anger lies a deeper layer of being hurt. We often carry a wound because our needs were not met adequately earlier on in life. So we need to become more conscious of our feelings and take responsibility for them. The first step is to acknowledge the feeling of anger and take charge of it. The second step is to recognize its cause, and the third is to address it. If there are a lot of unconscious emotions bubbling up to the surface, we need to find a way of dealing with them and there are special meditation practices that can allow you to express these feelings (see, for example, Dynamic Meditation, pp.64-7). Do not feel guilty about feeling angry. We need to give ourselves permission to release these feelings and not hold them in.

For a meditator it is possible to watch emotions without repressing them. This is only possible if the watcher within (see also p.47 and pp.94-5) has become strong enough and through daily meditation this can happen. Firstly, you are able to watch your body sensations, pleasure, and pain; secondly, you learn to watch your thoughts; and thirdly, you become able to watch the more subtle layers of emotion.

You are not your feelings: you create distance between yourself and them. There is a danger here that you may think you are watching your feelings, and you are indeed in control of them, though you are repressing them. Doing this constantly can create illness over time and to avoid this you need to learn to respect and understand yourself better. It is important to connect with yourself and love yourself. The more you love yourself the more easily you can let go of anger and other negative emotions. There is nothing wrong with experiencing anger and intense emotions; they are energies that keep us moving. But if we become aware of them and do not hold them back, we will feel more healthy and alive.

When the Russian mystic Gurdjieff was a child, his dying father told him a secret about life, not really expecting the boy to understand what he meant. He whispered in his ear, "Whenever you are angry because of someone else, wait for twenty-four hours before you act. If you still feel angry go to the person and tell them what you need to say." Gurdjieff did not understand this but tried to remember the words. Later, as an adult, he followed his father's advice and realized that typically, when he felt very angry, his anger disappeared within a few hours. Then after twenty-four hours he was able to see the other person's point of view, and sometimes even felt that the person was right. If he still thought the person was wrong after twenty-four hours, he went to talk to them about it.

The Stop Exercise

This exercise will increase your awareness and your mindfulness during physical activities. To become mindful while you are active helps you to stay in the present moment with whatever you are doing.

Integrate this exercise into your daily activities. If, for example, you are doing the washing-up, whenever you think of it, say, "Stop" out loud. Then stop whatever you are doing totally and do not move at all. After about 30 seconds, continue with what you were doing. Do this at least six times a day, or as often as you like.

2. "JUST FOR TODAY, DO NOT WORRY"

"Just for today, thou shalt not worry".
The second principle is intended to let us look into worrying. Where does worrying come from? Worry is a thought pattern that ultimately results from a feeling of being separate from others and from the universal whole. Worry is a negative belief system that prevents us trusting ourselves and the whole of existence. We worry that things may go wrong in the future, and we worry about things that went wrong in the past.

If you regret a past experience in your life, then learn the lesson you need to learn from it and move on. Worrying about the future is a futile activity, since it is always an unknown, and this scares us. Most of us want life to be secure, but in its very essence it cannot be. This makes every moment new and fresh, exciting, unpredictable, and adventurous. Trust yourself, trust life, and know that you are loved by God and life itself. This will let you surrender to events in your life, knowing that in the end everything will work out for the best. Even if at times things are unpleasant or unwelcome, later you will realize that an important experience took place.

Worrying creates tension and stress in body and mind. If we become aware that we are worrying, the next step is to see that there is nothing to be gained by it. It is not worth worrying about the past because it has already gone, and it is not worth worrying about future events because they may never happen. As soon as we realize that worrying never helps any issue or situation, we can drop it, like an old habit. If we worry a great deal, we are disconnecting ourselves from the present moment and from ourselves. We are not actively trusting ourselves or the process of life. Through Reiki, meditation practices, and prayer we learn to reconnect with our divine inner being .

3. "EARN YOUR LIVING HONESTLY"

"Earn thy living with honest labour".
The deeper meaning of this principle is about being honest with yourself. To be aware of your feelings, your longings, your values, and beliefs in life, and last but not least to realize who you truly are – a divine being. To live in truth means to be aligned to your Higher Self, to seek out clarity and guidance in life.

Being honest in your work includes doing what you want to be doing. Enjoy your work and carry it out as well as you can. Then you will love and respect yourself. If you have a job that you do not like, in the long term you harm yourself, perhaps even falling ill.

If you are honest with yourself then you are more likely to be honest with others. Honesty brings clarity and can activate deep encounters with others. This is an important part of life, in which we grow and learn from one another.

Having the sincere desire to seek out truth in each moment, we can see what projections we are placing on others. Repossessing our projections and owning them as our own wounds or unfulfilled desires, we can look closely at our lives and acknowledge with honesty where we are. In this way, relationships grow in depth and intimacy, with mutual valuing and respecting.

To live your life true to yourself needs courage. This means standing up for yourself, and stopping people from using you. In this way you come to recognize your own value and you start to love and respect yourself.

4. "HONOUR YOUR TEACHERS, PARENTS, AND ELDERS"

"Be kind to thy neighbours".
Reiki is the energy of unconditional love. We know that we all come from the same source and that there are only different expressions of forms and levels of energy vibration. Any positive energy directed to ourselves or others helps to heal. In a way we are all teachers and students of one another as we grow up. We share experiences with each other, we learn, we love, and we support each other. This principle is about letting every situation in life teach you something.

A great Sufi mystic, Hasan, was dying. One of his disciples asked him who his Master was. "I had many," said Hasan, "my Master was a dog. I was going to the river, thirsty, and a dog came along. He was also thirsty. As he looked into the river, he saw another dog there and became very afraid. He barked and ran away, but his thirst was so great that he returned. Eventually, despite his fear, he jumped into the water and the other dog vanished. At that moment I knew that a message had come from God: you have to jump in spite of your fears."

We learn so much from our parents and teachers. Even if we do not always agree with our parents' actions, we can be aware that they were in turn influenced by their own parents. Instead of blaming them we can think of them with understanding and compassion and show gratitude for all the good they have done on our behalf. To care about them, to love and respect them is to honour them in the right way.

5. "SHOW GRATITUDE TO ALL LIVING THINGS"

"Be thankful for the many blessings". Before giving a Reiki treatment we can say a prayer or a thank-you to life itself for being used as a channel for healing. We are not separate from other living beings but interconnected through Universal Life Energy – humans, animals, and plants. Being aware of this, we allow compassion and love to come into our lives. This is what gratitude means. It is another form of love, compassion, and respect for one another.

In this day and age we tend to take so much for granted, but there are many things in life, both big and small, to be grateful for: our own body, our health, good food, the beauty of nature, or the joy of a child. If we become more aware of how precious and spontaneous life is, we can appreciate situations as gifts from God. We can appreciate life itself and existence; and we can feel grateful for each new event in the sense of "Thy will be done". Then the whole of life becomes a prayer.

CONTEMPLATION OF THE REIKI PRINCIPLES

When you do this exercise you will gain more clarity and insight about each of the principles. You will also become more aware of how you can integrate them into your daily life. Do the exercise for about 15 minutes, or longer if you wish. Repeat this exercise on different days, for each Reiki principle.

Step one

Find a quiet place and make yourself comfortable. Spend a few moments relaxing yourself. Have a pen and paper, or your journal, nearby. Choose one of the principles to explore.

Step two

Close your eyes. Allow thoughts and feelings you have about your chosen principle to arise. What does the principle mean to you? Write you thoughts down.

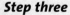

Step three

Speak the principle out loud and continue to write down your thoughts and feelings.

Step four

Now sit still and thank your unconscious mind for its co-operation. Don't judge your own thoughts or feelings about a principle.

The Gayatri Mantra

The Gayatri mantra is one of the most ancient mantras on earth. Its origin is unknown, but it is said that wisdom is contained within the powerful Sanskrit syllables of the Gayatri and that knowledge of the whole of life is born in this mantra.

THE EFFECTS OF THE GAYATRI MANTRA

The chanting of the Gayatri Mantra is intended to help us realize this truth, purifying the chanter as well as the listener. During the enunciation of the syllables vibrations of different frequencies and wavelengths are produced. There may be a calming of the chanter's nervous system, and a charging of the electrons in the body's energetic field. Over time, a subtle transformation is created in the chanter through a powerful awakening process. And with ongoing and sincere practice of the mantra there is the potential for the purification of thoughts and emotions, inner peace, clarity, experiencing of the divine in oneself and in others.

The mantra also transmits energy. This spreads and influences the consciousness of all to know enlightened awareness within.

As a spiritual practice the mantra is normally chanted 108 times, but if this is not possible, multiples of nine are recommended.

CHANTING THE GAYATRI MANTRA

◆ Sit alone or, better, in a group and start singing the Sanskrit words of the mantra.
◆ If the mantra is new to you, have the words in front of you and read them out a few times before you start.
◆ Either play the tape or ask an experienced chanter to start off the singing. Join in gradually and clap hands or use percussion instruments if you wish.
◆ Let yourself "get drunk" by the higher vibration of energy created by the energy of the mantra. Take in the spirit of it; purification of thoughts and feelings, inner peace, clarity, and the experience of the Divine in yourself.
◆ Let your body become loose. Sway to the rhythm of the chanting or move your body as you like.
◆ After twenty or thirty minutes stop chanting and sit silently for another ten minutes and feel the effects sink in.

"When you chant the Gayatri Mantra, it is a total offering. The frequency of the Gayatri Mantra purifies the atmosphere."

Shanti Mayi, contemporary realized Master

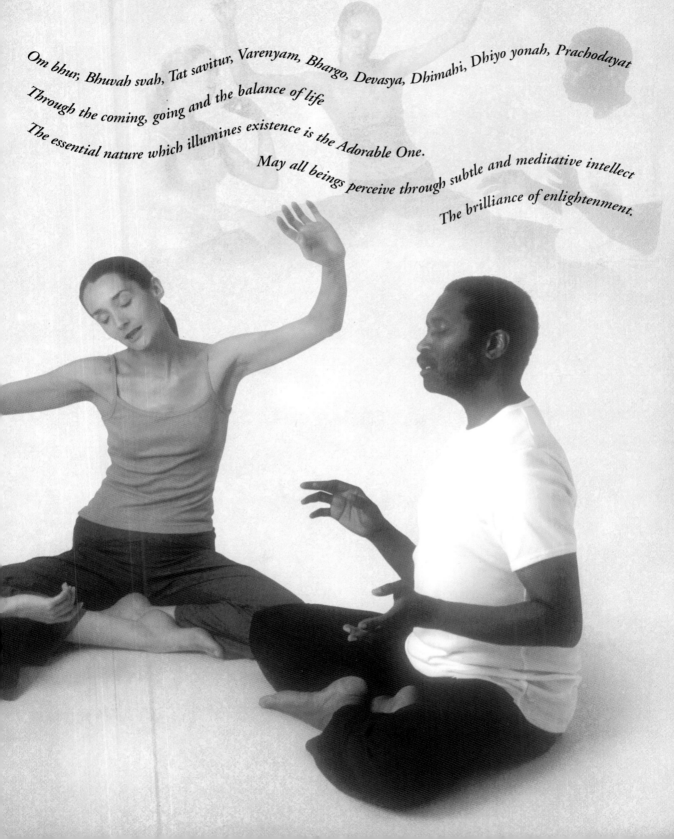

Om bhur, Bhuvah svah, Tat savitur, Varenyam, Bhargo, Devasya, Dhimahi, Dhiyo yonah, Prachodayat

Through the coming, going and the balance of life

The essential nature which illumines existence is the Adorable One.

May all beings perceive through subtle and meditative intellect

The brilliance of enlightenment.

Using the Reiki Symbols

Symbols and mantras are ancient tools used by humans to communicate with each other. Over the course of time the use of symbols disappeared from daily life and were mainly used in religious ceremonies. The sound of the mantra and the pictorial drawing of the symbol create a certain vibration of energy. For example, in the Reiki attunement process the Reiki Master uses symbols and mantras. These are needed to open the receiver's own inner healing channel, to amplify the flow of energy and let more Universal Life Energy flow through the upper energy centres (chakras). Sounds and mantras together have the ability to vibrate certain chakras. Through repetition of a mantra (for example "AUM", see p.100), you can activate the upper energy centres.

The Reiki symbols and their mantras are confidential and are only passed on to students of the Second and Master degree. They are therefore not published in this book.

THE ATTUNEMENT PROCESS

The Reiki attunement process is different from any other hands-on healing methods, transmitting energy to the student in an amplified state. It is an ancient technique that creates an open channel for cosmic energy to flow into the top of the student's head, through the upper body and out through the hands. In this process the vibratory level of the body is amplified. The physical body takes several weeks to adjust to the new level of energy vibration and a deep cleansing process on the physical, mental, emotional, and spiritual levels takes place.

SUPPRESSED EMOTIONS

After receiving Reiki attunements students tend to feel emotions rising to the surface and this is normal and to be expected. Issues that had been bubbling away, and possibly suppressed, often make themselves known. Whatever wants to be healed has to surface and be exposed. It is important to acknowledge these emotions, sometimes through expressing them and then letting go of them, and certain meditation techniques help to release emotions and then ground them.

"I feel more centred, peaceful, calm, more intuitive, learning to trust my intuition more. I don't worry so much, I tend to go with the flow of events in my life. I am more gentle with myself and I've learned to say 'No' more easily and not to feel guilty about it. I feel far more in control of my life. Since my initiation I have realized how much better I am in not letting others enter my space so much and how much stronger I have been in crises."

Dorothy

" I experienced a feeling of calm, total relaxation, deep heat and tingling through the hands. It was a time to clear and calm a busy head and allow a sense of relaxation to sweep over me. A few hours later I experienced a renewed sense of vigour and lots of energy and enthusiasm for life."

Jean

"Whenever I lie down to treat myself my cat jumps on to my chest and sits very, very still for about ten minutes. He too wants Reiki!"

Susan

The First Reiki Symbol

The First Reiki Symbol activates and increases the general available energy. It is used wherever energy is lacking – for example, in body treatment. If we use the First Symbol for certain areas of the physical body, it stimulates and purifies the energy in this part of the body. The vibration of the Symbol immediately affects the etheric body (see pp.20-1). Having applied the First Symbol to the body, this part starts to vibrate at a higher frequency and releases toxins from the physical body. Generally, the First Symbol stimulates a natural and harmonious flow of energy throughout the body.

CHARGING AND CLEANSING

The First Symbol can also be used to charge and cleanse objects and rooms – for example, for overnight stays in hotel rooms or for cleansing your crystals. It is also good to cleanse your treatment room before and after a Reiki healing session and to fill it with the purifying vibration of the First Symbol. To enrich your food apply the First Symbol while preparing your meal, holding your hands over the food for a while. If you eat out in restaurants you can change the vibration of the food and cleanse it by using the First Symbol. The Symbol also protects against outside energies – for example, at public events, or while travelling in buses and trains. We can visualize the symbol in front of us and energetically construct a protective screen.

USING THE SYMBOL

By using the First Symbol we can enhance our awareness and get in touch with our inner centre. Whenever you want to centre yourself, such as before giving a Reiki treatment, before meditating, or whenever you want to gain clarity about an issue in your life, such as before making an important phone call or making a big decision, try the exercise on these pages.

When you have finished the exercise, rest in your own centre and be open to any messages and insights that come. From this resting point you can come forward and take necessary action in the right frame of mind and body.

EXERCISE TO ENHANCE AWARENESS AND GAIN CLARITY

Apply the First Reiki Symbol.

Step one

Sit comfortably and take a few deep breaths. With each out-breath let go of thoughts and tension in the body. After a few minutes you will feel more relaxed.

Step two

Place your hands on your cheekbones, covering your eyes, and give yourself Reiki for a couple of minutes. Relax.

Step three

Now raise your hands in front of you and draw the First Symbol. Visualize it in golden light and say the mantra of the Symbol three times. Continue holding your hands in front of you. Feel the energy and vibration of the Symbol emanating from your palms. Continue holding your hands like this for 3 to 5 minutes. Feel the vibration of the Symbol and allow the radiating energy to reach your own centre. This level of vibration activates your awareness and helps you become clearer about things. It will also connect you more strongly with your own centre.

The Second Reiki Symbol

The Second Reiki Symbol adds a quality of harmony, peace, and balance to the etheric body and its chakras. This symbol is used especially for Mental Healing, making connection between the three layers of the mind: the conscious, the subconscious, and superconscious mind, known as the Higher Self.

HIDDEN REGIONS

The giver makes contact, using the Reiki symbols, with these hidden regions of consciousness and can receive messages and knowledge about the cause of illnesses and other problems. Fears, addictions, and other mental disturbances can be influenced positively. Mental Healing offers an opportunity to gain more awareness about past conditioning and programming, and it encourages you to seek more clarity in your life. This is an important step toward healing.

You can also give yourself Mental Healing. By doing so you deepen your connection with your own subconscious and Higher Self. A good time to do this is in the morning, when you have just woken up or at night before you go to sleep.

QUALITIES AND USES

The relaxing and calming quality of the Second Symbol is important. We can apply it to the physical body – for example, to areas that are over-stimulated. The vibration of the Second Symbol is absorbed by the etheric body and loosens up blocked energy. This supports the body's natural flow of energy and balances it. If there is a serious imbalance in the flow of energy, we need to apply the Symbol and give Reiki for at least three days in a row.

We can also use the Second Symbol to harmonize the quality of energy in a room. For example, after a party or a get-together with friends, with plenty of conversation, we can apply the Second Symbol and balance and calm the rotating energy. After a full day of mental activity we might want to calm down and be quiet. Here we can use the Second Symbol to balance and harmonize our own energy.

REIKI MENTAL HEALING

This technique is done only by those who have received the Second Degree Reiki training and the confidential Reiki Symbols. Actual procedure is taught by certified Reiki Master–Teachers in the Second Degree.

Mental Healing is a special method for dealing with deeply emotionally rooted and mental problems. The technique allows you to contact the unconscious and the superconscious, or the Higher Self, and to bring about healing in the receiver via the Spirit. This is used to address problems such as sleeplessness, addictions (compulsive alcohol abuse, eating disorders, smoking, and drug abuse), depression, or nervousness.

You can also use Mental Healing to become aware of any hidden reason for an ongoing issue, problem, or illness in your life. Part of the healing is to contact the unconscious mind and ask, "What is the reason underlying this problem?" Name the problem or issue, as in, for example, "my bladder infection" and ask the superconscious mind, "What must I do to become healthy again?"

BRINGING UNDERSTANDING

By contacting the unconscious and superconscious of a person we can bring an understanding into the conscious mind. Through questions such as, "What is the belief system or experience beneath this issue?" the conscious mind can receive these messages, either from the unconscious or the superconscious via the conscious mind.

EXERCISE TO BALANCE AND HARMONIZE ENERGIES

Apply the Second Reiki Symbol. A good time to do this exercise is just before going to sleep.

Step one

Sit or lie comfortably and relax. Draw the Second Symbol over the back of the head. Visualize it in a golden light and repeat the mantra of the Second Symbol three times.

Step two

Place your right hand on top of the head and your left hand in the medulla oblongata *area, where neck and head join. Hold your hands for five minutes and let the Reiki energy flow. Relax and feel the calming effect of the Second Symbol.*

The Third Reiki Symbol

The Third Reiki Symbol works on the mental level. It opens up intuition and strengthens the ability to "see". It is connected to the third eye (sixth) chakra and is used in Distant Healing, when healing energy and thoughts are sent on a mental level to people who are physically absent. Mental energy is vibration, which is normally sent in an unconscious way. For example, when we worry about someone or are angry with a person, he or she is receiving the thoughts and energy behind it, without being aware that anyone is thinking angrily about them.

With the Third Symbol we can use this ability to send energy and thoughts on a mental level consciously and send loving thoughts and healing energy to people. The Third Symbol affects the third eye of the giver and keeps in touch with the receiver's third eye. Communication happens on this high level of consciousness, which is in touch with the Higher Self of both giver and receiver.

BRIDGE OF LIGHT

During Distant Healing we create a transmission of healing energy to the receiver as if "over a bridge of light", transferring vital energy over long distances. The healing power is amplified during Distant Healing because mental forces are very strong. The giver senses distinctly the different flows of energy moving into the various parts of the receiver's body. If you do not know the receiver, a photograph may help visualize and focus the healing energy.

With Distant Healing you can send healing energy and light to people, animals, plants, and problem areas such as disasters and war zones. You can even send thoughts of peace and healing to flow to the whole planet. Reiki Distant Healing is a wonderful way to bring relaxation, awareness, and light to a dying person, especially if you personally cannot be present at the time. This is a unique way for you to say goodbye to the departing person.

ASKING PERMISSION

At the beginning of your Distant Healing always ask the person whether they want to receive healing from you. Then wait for the answer to come. Never carry out a treatment against someone's will. The best advice is to wait until you are asked before you send Reiki. You can also send yourself Distant Healing at any time. The exact procedure for Distant Healing is taught by a Reiki Master during Second Degree training.

EXERCISE TO SEND ENERGY OVER A DISTANCE

Before sending Distant Healing make an appointment with your receiver, if possible.

Step one

Think of the receiver and get a clear mental image of them. Greet the person and ask whether he/she wants to receive healing.

Step two

If you are a Second Degree trainee use the First and Third Symbols and send Reiki healing energy. If not, think of something you want the person to receive. For example, a positive or loving thought such as, "I love and trust you. You are a lovable and valuable person." Or just send love and light. Send this healing energy on a mental level for 5 to 10 minutes.

Step three

To end your healing say, "Can I do anything else for you?" Then wait. If you receive an answer, see what it is, and if necessary continue the healing. Send love and light again and thank the person for receiving the healing. Now say goodbye and finish your healing by rubbing your hands together to break the connection.

The Fourth Reiki Symbol

The Fourth, or Master, Symbol strengthens the ability to open up to higher energies and to become a channel for them. The vibration, a gentle, pulsing energy, of this Symbol is a very strong force and is used by the Reiki Master to channel higher energies during the attunement process. The Symbol can be used for personal development and for meditation. The vibration of this symbol has a strong positive force. It should only be available to those who are seriously committed to healing, truth, compassion, and meditation.

DEVELOPING A DEEPER SENSE

It is important for each Reiki Master to sit and meditate with the Fourth Symbol, so that he or she can activate and feel the vibration of the symbol inside. This helps understanding of the deeper sense of Reiki healing, bringing the giver into contact with the higher energies and helping him or her more easily to open up to channel higher energies and to become at one with them.

SUPPORTING SPIRITUAL GROWTH

The use of the Master Symbol supports our own spiritual growth. We need to focus on the most important thing in life: our self-realization, to get to the bottom of who we truly are. To truly be a Master, we need to realize our own perfection. True Masterhood means to be in a state of light, wisdom, and knowing. We have moved beyond personality and negative belief programmes. Seeking our inner light and truth, each of us is on a spiritual journey, on our own path toward realization to recognize who we are.

MEDITATION WITH THE FOURTH SYMBOL

Apply the Fourth, or Master, Symbol.

Step one

Sit in a relaxed position on a chair or on the floor. Hold your spine straight, your shoulders relaxed, and have your eyes closed. Your hands can rest in your lap or on your upper legs.

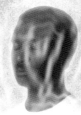

Step two

Now concentrate on your third eye (sixth chakra), between the eyebrows. Visualize or draw the Fourth Symbol with your third eye. Visualize it in golden light and say the mantra of the Symbol three times. Or, visualize the Fourth Symbol in golden light over the top of your head (crown chakra) and allow it to enter and flow into the entire body. Say the mantra three times.

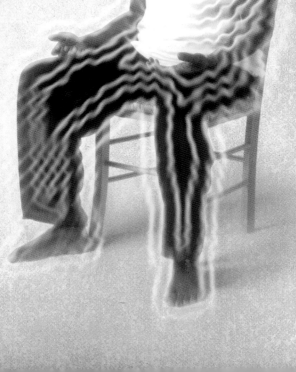

Step three

Feel the vibration of the Symbol and notice how it affects you. Sit and meditate with this Symbol as long as you like.

Epilogue

We all long to live in a better world: of peace, understanding, and harmony. There is chaos, war, and suffering in many places and often a situation has to get worse before it can get better. In order to cope with this we need to find an inner centre of peace within ourselves. From this place we may then begin to expand and share our understanding, love, and inner resources.

The intention of this book has been to support you in your own journey towards health and wholeness within. All the Reiki exercises and meditation techniques are helpful tools to heal and nourish you, and to explore who you really are. From this a deep relaxation, understanding, and conscious awareness arise about yourself and life itself. You are better able to enjoy life and to truly love and accept yourself. Once you love yourself, it becomes easier to love others.

Loving ourselves means we take responsibility for our lives and are able to heal ourselves. Learning that fear and misunderstanding are the root causes of most of our illness, distress, and suffering, we start to replace hatred, prejudice, and distrust with love, a willingness to co-operate, and an openness about the new and unknown. We all need to learn how better to communicate our thoughts and feelings to those around us. If we leave important things unspoken, we constrict our vital life energy and create tension and stress. Honest communication is needed to gain clarity and depth in relationships. All the methods in this book guide you to explore and become more honest and truthful with yourself and others.

We are entering a period of spiritual fulfillment and personal transformation. A powerful force is at work, coming from a higher plane, which challenges and helps us humans realize who we truly are. More and more people are taking up meditation and are in touch with the inner guidance of their Higher Selves. This creates a tremendous energy for self-healing and well-being. We need first to heal ourselves before we can go out and heal others and the planet. The spiritual awakening of thousands, if not millions, of human beings will release a huge amount of energy of love and healing. This may then transform the planet into a place where humans can live and share their peace, love, joy, and harmony with each other.

We are the secrets of God's treasure.
We are an ocean full of pearls.
We are part of the moon
And extend down to the fish.
We are also the ones who sit
At the throne of the Kingdom.

Jelaluddin Rumi

Guides to meditation

In deep relaxation you journey into your inner world. You meet your inner healer and receive everything you need. Choose a painting from the following pages. (This meditation takes between 20 and 30 minutes.) Look at the picture and relax. Close your eyes and let the picture look at you. Allow the picture to come closer and enter your heart centre. Let it melt into your heart and become one with the picture. Visualize yourself entering the landscape or shape and let the picture come alive. Explore your inner world through the picture. See, feel, and hear the picture's story. Allow your inner healer to appear in the picture and receive everything you need, bringing harmony and contentment. Carry this feeling into your life. Come back slowly to normal consciousness and move and stretch.

(Magno Shavdia is a well-known painter in Georgia, Russia. His paintings are visions arriving out of meditation, deeply connected with the spiritual world. His work has been exhibited all around the world.)

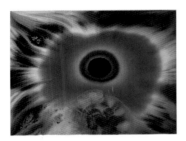

GIVING AND RECEIVING

"Stillness, a connection with myself, comfort, refreshment, hope, belief in myself; more trust with which to live life one day at a time without worrying about tomorrow, the day after, and the future." Sarah

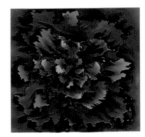

FIERY LEAVES

"Reiki brings peace and harmony to our busy, stressful lives. It allows a person to go within and experience a sense of calm and total relaxation. Reiki concentrates on positive energy to recharge our batteries." Jane

BLOSSOMING

"Reiki is my support – knowing it is always available is a great strength and I love the fulfillment I feel when giving Reiki to others. I really do feel it brings together mind, body, and spirit. It is a wonderful gift." Diana

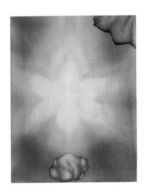

SAMASATI (RIGHT REMEMBRANCE)

"Reiki is a way for me to open myself as a channel, so the universal life force energy can flow into others, so they can then go on to heal themselves. It's about bringing clarity to chaos." Elaine

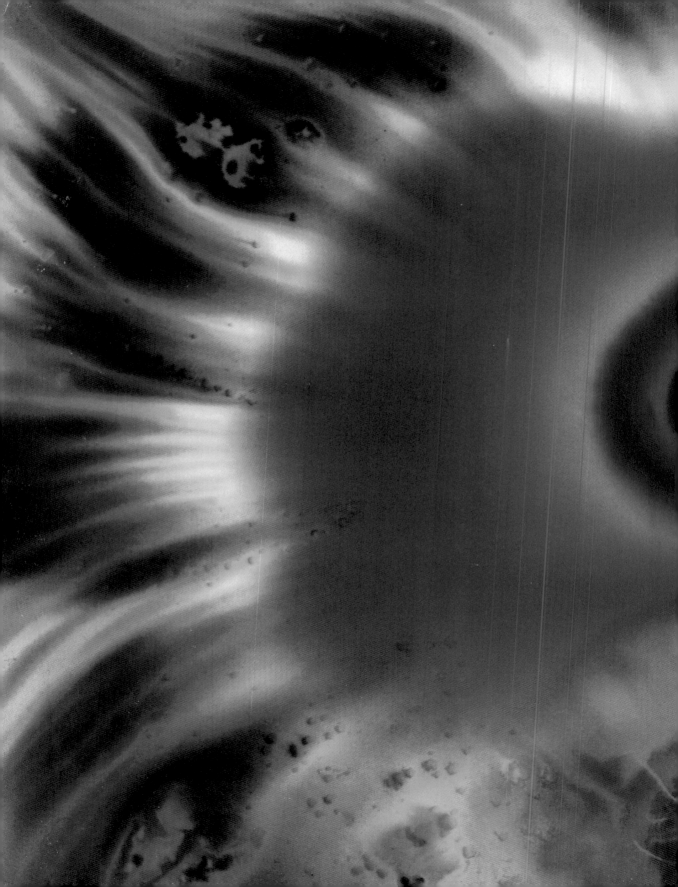

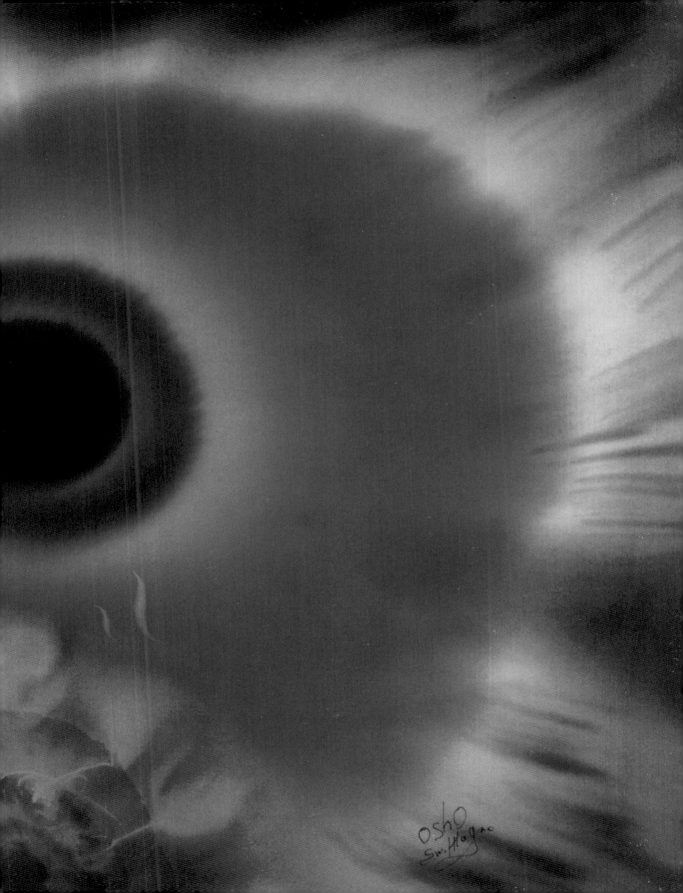

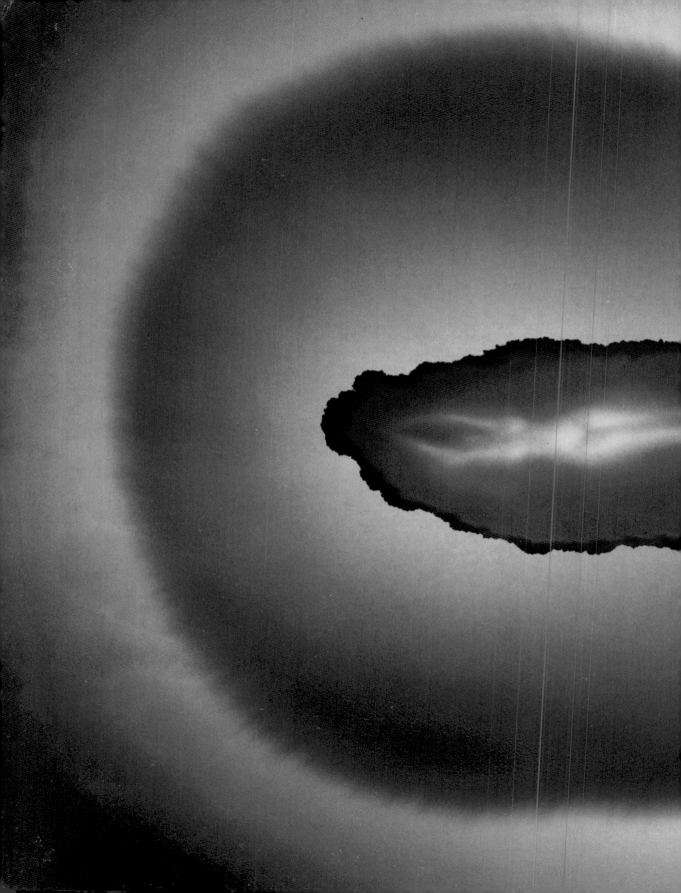

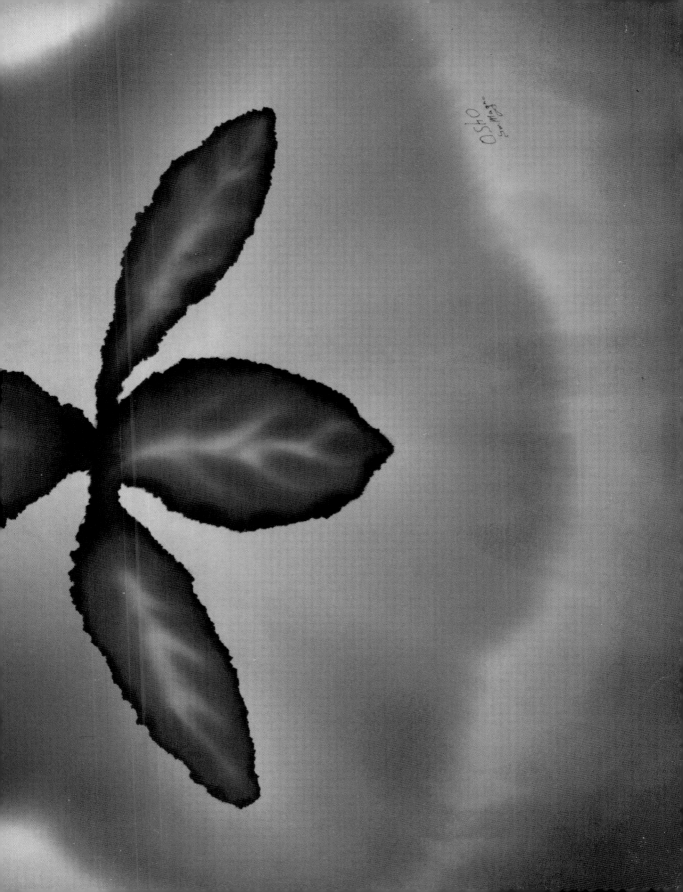

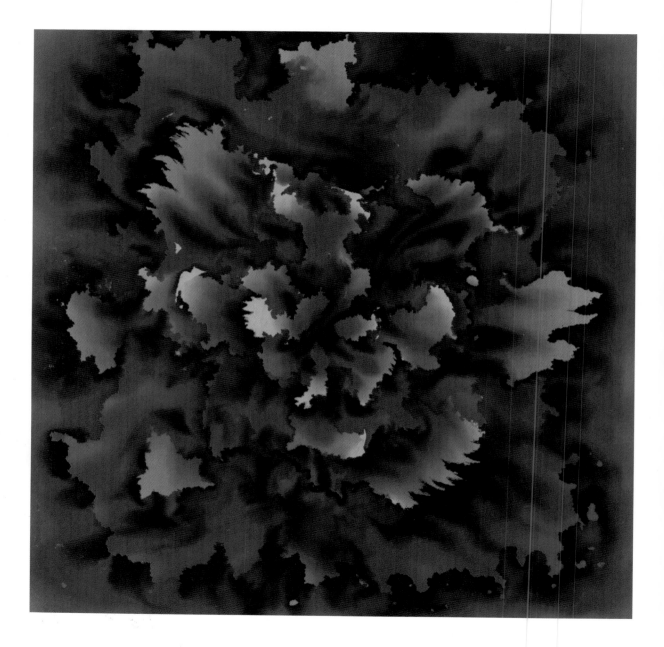

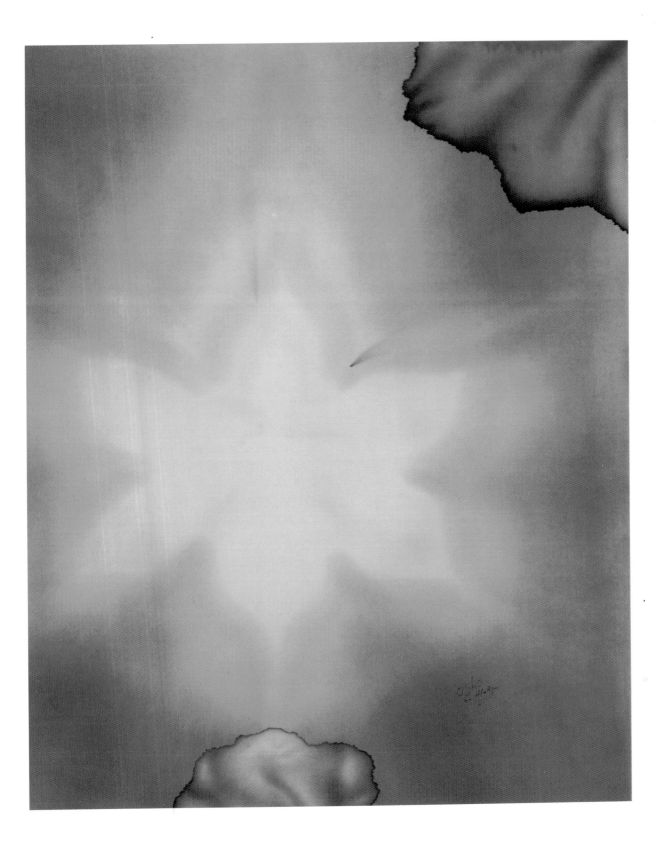

Glossary

Affirmation
A phrase or word describing a positive condition that we wish for ourselves.

Astral body
The fourth energy body associated with the heart chakra, the vehicle through which we love others.

Attunements
Special initiations in the Reiki energy, also known as energy transmissions. These open a channel for healing energies in the chakras.

Aura
The energy field surrounding the body; a subtle, invisible essence. The human aura can be rendered visible by Kirlian photography. The innermost etheric and emotional bodies are the easiest to discern.

Belief system
Beliefs that are established as we grow up, influencing our actions in life and opinions about ourselves and the world. Often we are unaware of them.

Centre
In meditation, this is the focal point of our consciousness, residing in the *hara*, or sacral chakra, allowing relaxation and nourishment from our inner source.

Chakra
Circular energy centre in the human subtle body. There are seven main chakras, located in the etheric body. In this book they are known as the root (first), sacral (second), solar plexus (third), heart (fourth), throat (fifth), third eye (sixth), and crown (seventh). The word "chakra" comes from the Sanskrit, meaning wheel. On the physical plane the chakras coincide approximately with the endocrine system.

Channel
An open vessel, allowing energy to flow through for the purpose of healing and higher consciousness.

Distant Healing
Allows you to send healing energies and thoughts on a mental level over a distance. Similar to radio and TV signals, healing energy is sent as though across a "golden bridge".

Divine
The force which can make us feel at one with each other and with all things.

Ego
The personality or Self in us, which makes us individual and separate from others.

Enlightenment
A state in which a person has experienced or lives his or her own divinity, and is awakened to truth and consciousness. It is a constant, permanent, selfless state.

Emotional body
The part of the body's energy field that lies between the etheric and mental bodies. It is related to our emotional state, the part of ourselves thought to be capable of separating from the physical body, as in dreaming or out-of-body experiences.

Etheric body
The energetic counterpart of the physical body, in which the chakras are located.

Existence
Life itself, or that which is referred to as God.

Gibberish
Nonsense language of spontaneous words used in

certain meditations so that the mind can be freed of conventional language and thought patterns.

Hara
A Japanese word for the sacral (second) chakra.

Higher Self
The part of us that is divine and gives us guidance – for example, in Mental Healing.

Incarnation
In Eastern religions and philosophies, people believe in more than one life in the physical form. After each death you are reborn until you have realized the truth and become enlightened.

Kirlian photography
A special method, developed by S. Kirlian in Russia, allowing the aura to become visible through photography.

Kundalini
Subtle energy considered to lie at the root chakra, which can rise up through the chakras, ultimately reaching the crown. Kundalini brings transformation at each chakra and enlightenment at the crown. Although liberating, its effects can be traumatic.

Leela
An Indian word meaning play. Often used to remind us that life is play.

Mantra
A word or a sound that sets subtle energies in vibration. They are used in meditations and in Reiki energy transmissions.

Meditation
A state of "not thinking" – "the awakening of the inner witness". Meditation happens in the present and is an immediate state of "not wanting, not doing". It is the ultimate state of relaxation.

Mental Healing
Healing through the mind by the emission of gathered mental energy. Can also take place in the form of Distant Healing.

Mystic
A being who lives in a state of enlightenment and *is* conscious awareness.

No-mind
The mind when it is in a state of "no thinking": no thoughts and no movement, in which "awakening" can happen.

Past life
See Incarnation.

Sanskrit
An ancient Indian language, the foundation of many modern languages. Hindu sacred texts are written in Sanskrit.

Spiritual Healing
The healer uses cosmic universal energy for treating the person. The only difference between it and Reiki is that in the Reiki technique a special attunement process is used to create higher vibrations in the student/giver.

Subtle body
The part of the body that is invisible to "normal" sight and charged with higher vibration – a layered energy field permeating and enveloping the physical body. It is thought to be composed of increasingly refined frequencies. The different bands of frequencies form the subtle bodies, each with differing properties, all essential for development and maintenance of a complete human being.

Glossary continued

Sufism
A group of seekers and mystics who originally came from Islam.

Superconsciousness
A level within us that is conscious and full of light, corresponding with the Higher Self, which knows and sees things clearly. Also known as intuition or spiritual guidance.

Symbols
A Symbol comprises a pictorial drawing and a name, or mantra. Reiki Symbols work on the body's healing channel, setting it in vibration, so increasing the vibrational frequency of the whole body.

Universal Life Force
The basic energy composing the whole manifest Universe and lying behind everything we are aware of. When it animates a living organism it becomes the life force.

Useful addresses

The Reiki Association
Cornbrook Bridge House
Cornbrook, Clee Hill, Ludlow
Shropshire, SY8 3Q
England
Tel./fax: 01584 891 197

The Reiki Alliance
PO Box 41
Cataldo ID 83810-1041
USA
Tel.: (208) 783-3535, fax: (208) 783-4848

Reiki Outreach International
PO Box 191156
San Diego
CA 92159-1156, USA
Tel/Fax: (619) 337-1500
www.annieo.com/reikioutreach

Mornington Peninsula Reiki Centre
10 Messines Road
Bittern 3918
Victoria
Australia
Tel.: 0359 83 9971

European Centre ROI
Jurgen Dotter
PO Box 326
D-83090 Bad Endorf
Germany
Tel./Fax: 08053 9242

Healing Academy
Clean Nishishinjuku Bldg.5F
7-5-6 Nishishinjuku
Shinjuku-ku, Tokyo 160-0023
Japan
Tel.: +81-3-3371-1644, Fax: +81-3-3371-1640

Bibliography

Blome, Goetz, *Mit Blumen heilen*, Bauer Verlag

Brennan, Barbara Ann, *Hands of Light*, Bantam, 1988

Brennan, Barbara Ann, *Light Emerging - The Journey of Personal Healing*, Bantam, 1993

Distel and Wellmann, Wolfgang, *Der Geist des Reiki*, Goldman Verlag, 1995

Gerber, Richard, *Vibrational Medicine*, Bear and Company, 1988

Hall, Judy, *The Art of Psychic Protection*, Findhorn Press, 1996

Honervogt, Tanmaya, *The Power of Reiki*, Owl Books, 1998

Horan, Paula, *Empowerment Through Reiki*, Lotus Press, 1998

Long, Barry, *The Way In*, Long Books, 2000

Myss, Caroline, *Anatomy of the Spirit*, Bantam, 1997

Osho, *The Everyday Meditator*, Boxtree, 1993

Osho, *From Medication to Meditation*, C.W. Daniel Company, 1994

Osho, *Meditation, the First and Last Freedom*, The Rebel Publishing House, 1995

Osho, *The Orange Book*, Rajneesh Foundation International, 1983

Petter, Frank Arjava, *Reiki Fire*, Lotus Press, 1998

Rumi, Mevlana Celaleddin, *Crazy As We Are*, Hohm Press, 1992

Zopf, Regine, *Das Unsichtbare wird sichtbar, Die Chakren und ihre Bedeutung fuer den heutigen Menschen*, Weltenhueter Verlag, 1998

Zopf, Regine, *Das Unsichtbare wird sichtbar, Die Energiekoerper des heutigen Menschen*, Weltenhueter Verlag, 1993

Zopf, Regine, *Reiki - Ein Weg sich selbst zu vervollkommen*, Weltenhueter Verlag, 1995

Meditation and Reiki music

Meditation music for many of the techniques described in this book and special Reiki music, as well as Tanmaya's tape, *A Guided Self-Treatment*, and CD, *Heal Yourself with Reiki* (in English and German), are available through the School of Usui Reiki, PO Box 2, Chulmleigh, Devon EX18 7SS, tel. +44 (0) 1769-580899.

For more information about Reiki in general, its history, Reiki degrees, basic Reiki hand positions, a short treatment form, harmonizing the chakras, Reiki for everyday stress, mental healing, and distant healing see Tanmaya's first book, *The Power of Reiki*.

Index

AUTHOR'S ACKNOWLEDGEMENTS

I want to thank Osho for making my life so much richer. The wisdom and abundance I have received from him flows throughout the book. I would like to thank Peter Campbell for his creative ideas and support. Thanks to Jo Godfrey Wood for editing the text. Many thanks to all my Reiki students who have shared their healing experiences and allowed me to use their comments on Reiki. Thanks to Osho International Foundation, New York, for allowing me to use Osho's words and meditation techniques in this book. I want to thank Magno Shavdia for providing his beautiful paintings and letting me use them for healing meditations in this book.

PUBLISHER'S ACKNOWLEDGEMENTS

Gaia Books would like to thank the following individuals and organisations for their help in the production of this book: Alex, Sharma, Dhyani, Ken, Caron, for modelling; Pip Morgan and Susanna Abbott for editorial help; Elizabeth Wiggans for indexing; The Osho International Foundation, PO Box 5235, New York 10150 for the use of Osho's words and meditation techniques, as originally featured in *The Everyday Meditator*, *The First and Last Freedom* and *The Orange Book*, by Osho. (Osho International: www.osho.com).